Contemporary Developments in
Adult and Young Adult Therapy

Contemporary Developments in Adult and Young Adult Therapy

THE WORK OF
THE TAVISTOCK AND PORTMAN CLINICS
VOLUME 1

Edited by
Alessandra Lemma

Foreword by
Matthew Patrick

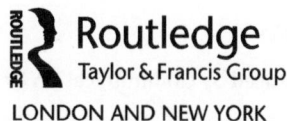

Routledge
Taylor & Francis Group

LONDON AND NEW YORK

First published 2012 by Karnac Books Ltd.

Published 2019 by Routledge
2 Park Square, Milton Park, Abingdon, Oxon OX14 4RN
52 Vanderbilt Avenue, New York, NY 10017, USA

Routledge is an imprint of the Taylor & Francis Group, an informa business

British Library Cataloguing in Publication Data

A C.I.P. for this book is available from the British Library

ISBN: 9781780490069 (pbk)

Edited, designed, and produced by Communication Crafts

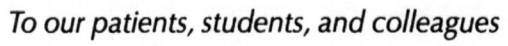
To our patients, students, and colleagues

CONTENTS

SERIES EDITOR'S PREFACE

Margot Waddell

Since it was founded in 1920, the Tavistock Clinic has developed a wide range of developmental approaches to mental health which have been strongly influenced by the ideas of psychoanalysis. It has also adopted systemic family therapy as a theoretical model and a clinical approach to family problems. The Clinic is now the largest training institution in Britain for mental health, providing postgraduate and qualifying courses in social work, psychology, psychiatry, and child, adolescent, and adult psychotherapy, as well as in nursing and primary care. It trains about 1,700 students each year in over 60 courses.

The Clinic's philosophy aims at promoting therapeutic methods in mental health. Its work is based on the clinical expertise that is also the basis of its consultancy and research activities. The aim of this Series is to make available to the reading public the clinical, theoretical, and research work that is most influential at the Tavistock Clinic. The Series sets out new approaches in the understanding and treatment of psychological disturbance in children, adolescents, and adults, both as individuals and in families.

In many ways, *Contemporary Developments in Adult and Young Adult Therapy*—the first volume in what will surely become known as "The Tavistock Trilogy"—succeeds in epitomizing aspects of the life and work of the two Clinics that comprise the Tavistock and Portman NHS Foundation Trust. Many of those who work here are often in two places at once: shouldering the ongoing challenges of the ever-changing clinical demands and requirements of people's troubled and troubling lives and, simultaneously, managing, administrating, and researching on an ongoing day-to-day basis. Yet at the same time, these clinicians are on the move in different parts of the country and the world—lecturing, teaching, and training.

Implicitly, this volume goes some way towards addressing how all this can be possible. An answer, of sorts, is that for so long this work culture has recognizably characterized, and belonged to, a commitment to a world of solid values: those of loyalty, cooperation, *esprit de corps*, and purpose—a culture that has a generous, moral, and informed spirit. Yet now we have to respond to a "new culture": the necessity to face the realities of the current political, economic, and cultural climate—the actuality of people's everyday lives in the midst of NHS changes and the exigencies and impositions of wider social pressures.

Different ways simply have to be found, ways that Alessandra Lemma's impressive collection of contributors, chapters, and ideas lays out with vigour. As she says, one of the central areas of the over-all Trust has always been the "developmental continuity" between childhood and adult mental difficulties. These will be further focused upon in the two subsequent volumes, where the emphasis will be on the depth of long-term psychoanalytic work and, differently, on the systemic model. One volume will address the complex dynam-ics between the internal and external worlds of children, adoles-cents, and their families; the other, the equally complex and related dynamic between the individual, the group, and institutional life. These subsequent two books will have their own style and emphasis, but I expect that among the many commonalities between all three will be a commitment to a pluralistic mental health context that can underpin the preservation of traditional principles. These volumes will look both ways: to the past as well as to the future. Indeed, such a perspective has been a familiar characteristic of the work of both Clinics since they were founded in the aftermath of the Great War. They were established in the face, respectively, of the fall-out from the casualties of war, shell-shock in particular, and of antisocial and delinquent behaviour—amidst, in other words, the countless fractured lives, loves, and losses of the time. The ongoing extreme mental and emotional work that these pages describe has, even now, much to do with those early initiatives.

This book does justice to the lessons of history but is also decisively modern—for it describes, with great precision, some of the ways in which the joys and privileges of innovative research survive and thrive in our times. In the present economically pressurizing culture, the nature of the external demands on, and deprivations of, both young people and adults has properly to be seen in relation to the long-recognized vicissitudes of the developmental picture: that the process of growing up, with all its problems of separation and individuation, is, significantly, how it has always been.

But one of the clear strengths of the thinking and clinical practice represented here lies in just how impressive some of the innovations and adaptations of more traditional work can be. The much more textured understanding of and cooperative creative integration with other services will enable new forms of growth. The reader is introduced to a range of research carried out by staff determined to maintain the best standards of practice.

The detail of the work, in so many individual, group, and community—and even online-based—settings, gives one hope that services will be able to expand and survive. Many of the chapters describe extremely testing situations, but they emphasize, above all, the importance of collaborative relationships. The book includes examples of both short- and long-term interventions, from forensic psychiatry to marital therapy and primary-care cooperation, as well as newly developing treatment models, from dynamic interpersonal therapy to the social media revolution. The engagement is with clinical need, on the one hand, and a cost-effective economy, on the other. One cannot but be impressed by the energy of writers who are struggling to keep internal and external worlds in relation to one another—which is the very essence of the work of both Clinics.

ACKNOWLEDGEMENTS

The idea for this book grew out of various discussions held within the Tavistock and Portman NHS Foundation Trust as part of our attempts to think about our work and our distinctive contribution to training and clinical services. Many people have therefore been involved in the thinking behind this series of three books, of which this is the first, each focusing on different aspects of the Trust's work in both the clinical and the training domains. In particular, I would like to thank Louise Lyon, Trust Director, and Matthew Patrick, Chief Executive, both of whom have always been very supportive of this project and have been involved in it in different ways. At the end of the day, this book would, of course, not have been possible without the enthusiastic and passionate engagement of all the contributors. I would like to thank them for agreeing to be involved. For me, it has been a pleasure and a privilege to edit this collection. I would also like to thank Klara King for her excellent copyediting, as ever, and Phillip Birch for all his help in getting the manuscript into its final form.

ABOUT THE EDITOR AND CONTRIBUTORS

Stephen Briggs has worked in the Adolescent Department at the Tavistock and Portman NHS Foundation Trust for 20 years and is currently the lead for the Psychodynamic Brief Therapy Service. He has written widely on adolescence, infancy, and suicide, including *Working with Adolescents and Young Adults: A Contemporary Psychodynamic Perspective* (2008), *Growth and Risk in Infancy* (1997), and *Relating to Suicide and Self Harm: Psychoanalytic Perspectives on Practice, Theory and Prevention* (2008, edited with Alessandra Lemma & William Crouch). He is Associate Dean, Specialist and Adult Mental Health Services, and Professor of Social Work and Director of the Centre for Social Work Research, Tavistock/University of East London.

Anca Carrington is a trainee psychotherapist in the Adult Department at the Tavistock Centre. She obtained her MA and PhD in economics, and, after nine years of university lecturing and research in this field, she joined the civil service, first as senior methodologist in spatial analysis at the Office for National Statistics, then as an economist at HM Treasury.

Andrew Cooper is Professor of Social Work at the Tavistock Centre and the University of East London. He has worked at the Tavistock since 1996 and is a former Dean of Post Graduate Training and the Director of Research and Development. He is a psychoanalytic psychotherapist working both in private practice and in the Adolescent Department. He has a long-standing interest in the psychoanalytic understanding of society and social processes. He coordinates the Tavistock Policy Seminar Series and currently has a role as public policy lead in the Trust.

Peter Fonagy is Freud Memorial Professor of Psychoanalysis and Head of the Research Department of Clinical, Educational and Health Psychology at University College London. He is Chief Executive of the Anna Freud Centre, London, and consultant to the Child and Family Programme at the Menninger Department of Psychiatry and Behavioural Sciences at the Baylor College of Medicine. He is also a Fellow of the British Academy.

Richard Graham is Clinical Director of the Adolescent Directorate of the Tavistock Clinic and is a consultant child and adolescent psychiatrist. After training in medicine and psychiatry in London, he specialized in adolescent psychiatry at the Tavistock Clinic and has continued to work there as a senior clinician and trainer. He is especially interested in contemporary issues for adolescents and adults, in the context of developments in media, technology, and the Internet.

Ellie Kavner is Head of Systemic Psychotherapy and a social worker at the Tavistock and Portman NHS Foundation Trust. She worked in statutory and voluntary sectors as a social worker and family therapist prior to this. Her clinical interests include the nature and consequences of intimate family violence and the impact of physical illness on families, and she has assessed and treated families involved in public and private legal proceedings. As a trainer she has participated in professional systemic therapist programmes and co-organized systemic management and leadership courses.

Alessandra Lemma is the Unit Director, Psychological Therapies Development Unit, Tavistock and Portman NHS Foundation Trust, and the Clinical Director of the Psychological Interventions Research Centre, University College London. She is a Fellow of the British Psychoanalytical Society. She is Visiting Professor, Psychoanalysis Unit, UCL, and Honorary Professor of Psychological Therapies at Essex

University, She is the Regional Editor (London) of the *International Journal of Psychoanalysis* and General Editor of the New Library of Psychoanalysis book series (Routledge). She has published several books and papers on psychotherapy, psychoanalysis, the body, and trauma.

Frank Lowe is a consultant social worker and psychoanalytic psychotherapist in the Adolescent Department of the Tavistock and Portman NHS Foundation Trust. He is the Head of the Young Black People's Consultation Service, teaches on a number of Tavistock courses, and has written several papers on race and psychotherapy.

Louise Lyon is Trust Director of the Tavistock and Portman NHS Foundation Trust. Previous positions within the Trust include Clinical Director of the Adolescent Department and Trust Head of Psychology. She is a clinical psychologist and adult psychoanalyst. In her clinical work she has specialized in working with adolescents and young adults. Before joining the Tavistock and Portman in 1996, she worked for over 10 years in the Psychology Department of the South Kensington and Chelsea Mental Health Centre. She has a long-standing interest in brief interventions and in supporting the development of pluralistic mental health services.

Carine Minne is a Consultant Psychiatrist in Forensic Psychotherapy at the Portman Clinic and Broadmoor Hospital, West London. She is the Training Programme Director for junior psychiatrist training in forensic psychotherapy between these two Trusts. She is a psychoanalyst at the British Psychoanalytical Society and chairs the Special Interest Group in Forensic Psychotherapy at the Royal College of Psychiatrists. One of her special interests is the provision of long-term psychotherapy for patients across the different levels of secure forensic psychiatry settings.

Matthew Patrick is the Chief Executive of the Tavistock and Portman NHS Foundation Trust and a training and supervising analyst for the British Psychoanalytical Society. Originally trained as an adult psychiatrist, for many years he combined clinical work and developmental research. His published work has focused on the development and nature of adult personality and personality disorders and the role of mental representation.

Brian Rock is a consultant clinical psychologist who completed his training in South Africa. Since 1996 he has worked in the NHS, largely in adult mental health, during which he completed the Tavistock adult psychoanalytic psychotherapy clinical training. He is a psychoanalyst with the British Psychoanalytical Society and is service lead for a new primary care service in City and Hackney linked to the Tavistock and Portman NHS Foundation Trust. His particular interest is the application of psychoanalysis in the NHS. He has completed training in Mentalization-Based Treatment (MBT) and is working towards accreditation as a Dynamic Interpersonal Training (DIT) practitioner/ supervisor.

Joanna Rosenthall was a senior staff member for over 20 years at the Tavistock Centre for Couple Relationships, where she ran the clinical training and Professional Doctorate programme in couple psycho-analytic psychotherapy. She now runs the Couples Unit in the Adult Department of the Tavistock and Portman NHS Foundation Trust. She also works with couples and individuals in private practice. She has published a number of papers in this area, recently focused on sex, couples who function as if fused, and violent couples. She is a member of the British Association of Psychotherapy and the British Society of Couple Psychotherapists and Counsellors.

Mary Target is a clinical psychologist and a psychoanalyst. She is Professor of Psychoanalysis in the Research Department of Clinical, Educational and Health Psychology at University College London. She is also Professional Director of the Anna Freud Centre. She is a Fellow of the British Psychoanalytical Society and Course Organiser of UCL's Masters Programme in Theoretical Psychoanalytic Studies, and Doctorate in Child and Adolescent Psychoanalytic Psychotherapy. She carries out research on child and adult attachment, personality functioning, and mentalization and has a part-time psychoanalytic practice.

Bernadette Wren trained as a Clinical Psychologist and Systemic Psychotherapist and is now Trust-wide Head of Psychology at the Tavistock and Portman NHS Foundation Trust. She teaches clinical research methods across a number of Tavistock courses and co-chairs the UEL–Tavistock Doctorate in Systemic Psychotherapy. She works clinically with transgendered young people and their families in the Trust's Gender Identity Development Service. She is currently involved in research focusing on parent–child communication, exploring a "social domains" model of family interactions.

Jessica Yakeley is a consultant psychiatrist in forensic psychotherapy at the Portman Clinic, and Director of Medical Education and Associate Medical Director of the Tavistock and Portman NHS Foundation Trust. She is also a Fellow of the British Psychoanalytical Society. She has a long-standing interest in medical education, has published papers on topics including psychodynamic teaching methods, risk assessment, MAPPA, prison health, and antisocial personality disorder, and is the author of *Working with Violence: A Contemporary Psychoanalytic Approach* (2010).

Linda Young is a consultant clinical psychologist and psychoanalyst working in the Adult and Adolescent Directorates of the Tavistock and Portman NHS Foundation Trust. She is current Head of the Tavistock Young People's Consultation Service, which is one service within the Tavistock Adolescent Department, for which she is also Clinical Lead. Her special interests include working with the aftermath of trauma, and interventions for young adults.

FOREWORD

Matthew Patrick
Chief Executive, Tavistock and Portman NHS Foundation Trust

Nature dictates that as individuals we are conceived, are born, and then at some point later die. The shape of the arc that we follow, involving growth and development with eventual decline, is something that we might all like to influence. It has been argued that the same basic curve is, however, followed by societies, civilizations, and, indeed, organizations. How does an organization influence its trajectory? How do organizations avoid the pull towards conservatism and protectionism associated with the developmental plateau found at the top of the curve? Organizations are living entities, made up of people and the relationships between them. How do *we* avoid becoming more inward-looking, more preoccupied with our own preferences and gratifications and less engaged with the world around us, and less irritated by constant demands for change?

I think that in this book Alessandra Lemma has given us something of an insight into this process within one organization, the Tavistock and Portman NHS Foundation Trust. One of the answers to emerge from these chapters is found in the passion, interest, and curiosity that the authors convey in the world around them, coupled with a quality of openness to the outside, alien or new. But the answer may also have to do with how an organization understands itself and its purpose and how it manages to integrate its history into its present.

Henry Dicks, writing about the first 50 years of the Tavistock Clinic, describes the origins of the organization:

> While psychodynamic, the Clinic's doctrine beyond this general orientation was to "have no doctrine", but only aims: to help, to understand more and to teach its work. As such it was the meeting-ground of psychotherapists of several schools or of none, making for a certain vagueness and lack of theoretical homogeneity, but also for flexibility and a wide variety of techniques and viewpoints. . . . Its image was always that of an open forum, of a synoptic viewpoint and ethically above reproach. [Dicks, 1970, p. 2]

Thus a focus on aims as opposed to dogma was central from the start. In addition, I think that the organization always sought to make a radical contribution as opposed to a conservative one. Such a contribution *demands* absolute engagement with the wider society, but also perhaps an uncomfortable positioning just on the edge of the establishment.

Maybe the capacity for self-renewal also has to do with an attitude towards development within ourselves. If our trajectory is not to follow a more basic arc, I think we have to support the creation of new branch points within ourselves—both as individuals and as organizations—and encourage the mavericks and entrepreneurs who will force such branching. We then need to support new branches through the provision of a trellis—a framework of ideas, values, and attitudes that encourages growth without seeking to exert excessive control. We also need to undertake the painful work of pruning. This is the work that goes on painfully in the background of any successful organization.

In content this book is not about pruning. It is, though, about developments and innovation and about the trelliswork of ideas that supports them and the core values from which they grow.

In bringing together this collection, Professor Lemma has undertaken the role of skilled gardener herself. The work of the Trust is now broad. Training and education makes up almost half of the activity and Child and Adolescent Mental Health Services over half of the clinical work. Professor Lemma has, in this first volume, broadly focused her attention on our work with adolescents and adults. She has selected the content carefully, paying as much attention to what is left out as to what is included. She has clearly selected her authors for their quality and supported them with similar care. All of this is evident in the chapters that comprise this book, and in the description of an organization struggling to evolve in a manner that links it inextricably to the communities and society within which it is situated as much as to its own history.

Now, in 2012, as an NHS Mental Health Trust, I think we see ourselves as a public benefit organization. Our vision is focused on the type of communities and society that we want to contribute to creating and to be a part of. The work represented here remains, I think, a radical contribution. It espouses a patient- and client-centred agenda that, at its heart, challenges the traditional medical model of mental health care; it involves the organization itself in relinquishing any view that it, or others like it, might hold a "master narrative" in relation to emotional and psychological health and illness. What I hope comes across is a wish to make a positive difference.

Beyond this, what is represented here is an organization rooted in ideas and in the innovative translation of them into effective practice—an organization seeking to contribute to the pool of ideas through research and development, but also committed to bringing together the best ideas of the time, old and new, from inside and out, together with the most gifted and able professionals in related fields of endeavour.

Working *alongside* has to be a key component of our organization's identity: aiming to work *in* the communities we serve, either as individuals or in teams, listening, learning, sharing, exchanging, and working *with* others as partners.

All of the work is characterized by a model of reflective practice that encourages open discussion, with a belief that this style of practice encourages awareness of the impact that the work has on all those involved, and helps develop resilience as well as competence.

The Tavistock and Portman NHS Foundation Trust is, however, a complex organization—as, indeed, are they all. We are perhaps more of a tribe than a family, a gathering together of like-minded people who also hold tenaciously to distinctive family identities. As such, relationships within the organization are not always easy, and one can feel this, I think, in the chapters contained herein: a sense of the struggle involved in the writing. Are the authors representing an organization, its history, and the generations who have contributed to it, are they representing their family beliefs and values, or are they representing their own ideas? It is perhaps because ultimately they choose the latter that the organization has continued to grow and to flourish—not without pain and loss, but also with much gained.

Reference

Dicks, H. V. (1970). *Fifty Years of the Tavistock Clinic*. London: Routledge & Kegan Paul.

PART I

AS WE ARE NOW

Introduction

Alessandra Lemma

The Tavistock—or "Tavi", as it is still referred to by many—is concretely as well as metaphorically "an institution". This "brick mother" (Rey, quoted in Steiner, 1994), now officially twinned with the Portman Clinic, acquires for all who engage with it a particular resonance. For some, it is a place that holds the promise of help and transformation; for others, it is a "special" training school or workplace that values reflective practice within broader public health and social care services; for yet others, it still remains the embodiment of a fossilized ivory tower. In truth, the Tavistock and Portman Clinics can be all these things some of the time and much more besides.

Whether it is viewed fondly or with suspicion, the Tavistock has a distinguished history in the development of psychoanalytic and systemic ideas and their application to the treatment of mental health problems. For me it is a privilege to be editing a book about therapeutic work with adults and young people that has developed within this particular institution, which is now called the Tavistock and Portman NHS Foundation Trust.[1]

Since the Tavistock Clinic was founded, in 1920, by Dr Hugh Crichton-Miller to help survivors of shell shock and the Portman

3

Clinic, in 1933, as the clinical arm of the Institute for the Study and Treatment of Delinquency, these clinics have established themselves nationally and internationally as landmarks in mental health care and training. Institutions become a canvas for many projections, and the Tavistock and Portman Clinics are no exception. In many people's minds they remain psychoanalytic institutions, and, as such, they have been criticized as being too inward-looking, offering primarily long-term psychoanalytic psychotherapy to a few, operating as if existing outside the exigencies of the "real" National Health Service. Like all projections, this has a kernel of truth in it, and as an institution we have had to grapple with the implications. But the kernel of truth is part of a bigger picture that is somewhat distorted by the projection—and, importantly, this is a picture that is constantly being updated as the institution engages with the external NHS context of which it is a part.

Indeed, a closer a look at this institution immediately exposes how diverse it actually is. For example, although the Tavistock Clinic has been home to a number of distinguished psychoanalytic thinkers, for many years it has also been the home of creative and influential systemic colleagues. Even within the psychoanalytic domain of its work, the idea that all it offers is long-term, open-ended psychotherapy has never been true of the work of the Adolescent Directorate, or the Trauma Service in the Adult Directorate, or the Under-Fives Service in the Child and Family Directorate, all of which have developed and have for many years now provided brief psychoanalytically informed interventions (e.g. Garland, 2002; in this volume, see chapter four, by Linda Young & Frank Lowe). But the long-term work provides a fundamental backbone to the development of the psychoanalytic applications described in this volume.

Nowadays the services and training offered by the Tavistock and Portman Clinics are responsive to the demands of a modern health-care economy. Many of its clinical services are provided in community settings, reaching a diverse group of patients whose psychiatric morbidity is high and whose external circumstances reflect social, economic, and emotional deprivation. Its training programmes also include colleagues who have no academic qualifications and many who are working on the front line in NHS or social care contexts.

The Portman Clinic has, from its inception, always focused on understanding and treating individuals whose violent and sexualized behaviour places them at the margins of society. Its clinical and research activity thus addresses the most disturbed and disturbing patients, and close links have been forged with several forensic services and prisons across the United Kingdom.

One of the aims of this volume is to capture the variety and richness of contemporary developments within the Tavistock and Portman Clinics as they pertain to work with adults and young adults. Two subsequent books, which will form part of a trilogy, will address, respectively, applications with children and their families and consultation.

The chapters in this book attempt to capture the collective voice as well as the highly individual voices that constitute the Tavistock and Portman Clinics at this particular juncture in their respective histories. In this Introduction I do not attempt to review the history, nor do I go over each chapter individually; rather, from the privileged position of having edited this collection, I want to draw out some overarching themes that have emerged and that connect with broader discourses relevant to the delivery of mental health care and the rewards and challenges of organizational life.

The chapters in Part I provide a meta-perspective from which to consider the applied work that follows. Part II is concerned with clinical applications, illustrating work with young adults, adults, and diverse patient groups (for example, chapter six, by Carine Minne, on work with forensic patients) delivered through different modalities (for example, chapter seven, by Joanna Rosenthall, on work with couples). Part III focuses on clinical and service innovations informed by a psychoanalytic understanding of the mind.

The task of editing a book about the work of an institution of which I am also a member has been challenging. Trying to do justice to the different theoretical traditions is not easy, given that I can only approach this task from my own vantage point: that of being a psychologist and a psychoanalyst. But even as a psychoanalyst I cannot claim to be representative of my psychoanalytic colleagues. All I can do is to take responsibility if I have misunderstood or misrepresented any of the traditions or disciplines that make up this institution. Inevitably, what I outline here is an attempt—as one voice among many—to capture my own version of some of the points of convergence and of some of the tensions that I perceive.

The final cause

The institution is united in a shared vision for improving mental health and emotional well-being, a vision that places its emphasis on "the importance we attach to social experience at all stages of people's lives. We are also distinct in our focus on psychological and developmental approaches to the promotion of health and the prevention and treatment of mental ill health".[2] But, as will become apparent on reading the three volumes that together aim to capture the work of this organization, what defines the Tavistock and Portman Clinics is a range of therapeutic approaches and modes of service delivery. In this volume the diversity at the level of intervention is less apparent, since much of the work with adults and young adults is primarily informed by psychoanalytic ideas, but even here diversity is the order of the day. This unity through diversity is an example of what Aristotle (Ross, 1950) referred to as the "final cause"[3]: "the end (telos), that for the sake of which a thing is done". In this instance the final cause is improving mental health and emotional well-being, and this alerts us to the fact that, in theory at least, different paths may lead to the same outcome (Lear, 2009). In other words, the final cause does not dictate which, among the ways of doing psychotherapy, is a right or a better way.

Three conceptual vertices—the developmental, relational, and social vertices—cut across the differences and inform clinical services and training activity.

The developmental vertex

The developmental model that informs the work is inherently relational, since it subscribes to a view that the mind develops in and through our relationships from birth onwards. It provides a framework for understanding the complex relationship between early experience, social environment, genetic inheritance, and psychopathology. Exciting progress has been made in understanding the interaction between our genetic constitution and our social environment, which allows genes either to manifest themselves in the phenotype or suppress them altogether. There is an increasingly strong evidence base to support the formative impact of early childhood relationships on adult personality and psychopathology. Adult mental health problems are developmental in nature; three quarters can be traced back to mental health difficulties in childhood, with 50% arising before the age of 14 years (Kim-Cohen et al., 2003). Prospectively, mental health problems experienced in childhood or adolescence are similarly often associated with serious difficulties in adult life, including enduring morbidity (Jenkins et al., 2008).

The developmental continuity between childhood difficulties and adult mental health problems is sobering, and it is a potent reminder of the vital importance of integrated services that can respond to the needs of families as well as those of individuals. It also underscores why we need to focus on preventative interventions that can help break otherwise repetitive cycles, often of an intergenerational nature.

The relational vertex

Different modes of therapy are represented in this Trust: individual, couple, family, and organizational/group. The way the therapy or consultation is delivered thus looks very different—you can literally count the differences depending on how many people come together in the same room to work on a "problem". What is striking, however, is that irrespective of the differences in how the intervention is delivered or its theoretical home, the consistent emphasis throughout all of the chapters is on the importance of understanding the individual in the context of the matrix of his or her relationships: the relational vertex. In this sense we could say that there is no such thing as "individual" work, because even the individual therapist keeps in mind and works with the full constellation of the patient's relationships, internal and external. There is also no such thing as an "individual" problem that does not also in some way tell the story of a relationship or sets of relationships, often across several generations (Faimberg, 2005).

Both systemic and psychoanalytic therapists prioritize this relational domain as their focus of intervention: whether the patient presents individually or in a couple or family, these interventions approach the presenting problem as a communication about relationships, about the referred patients' internal and external interpersonal worlds. This is a distinctive hallmark of the psychological interventions offered within this institution. Here the similarities end, however: beliefs about how relationships shape the mind, the extent to which actual versus phantasized relationships have the upper hand in the aetiology of mental health problems, and what kinds of techniques help people to be freed of destructive ties to others distinguish these modalities—indeed, even the language we use to refer to what we do will differ.

Psychoanalytic approaches, which inform all the chapters in this book, alight on the unconscious dimensions of the relational vertex: the fabric of the internal world comprises multiple, often conflicting, unconscious representations of self-with-others. They focus on the way our current relationships are informed by developmental models that have not been "updated". Systemic approaches cast the net wider and seek to take into account the meaning and impact on the individual of broader systems, those of the actual family and of the wider social and cultural group, bringing into focus the intricate networks of external relationships that shape the individual.

These different perspectives[4] engage us passionately. Yet the passion with which we relate to our beliefs is not evidence that we have access to any kind of ultimate truth. Indeed, empirical evidence suggests, for example, that there are many effective therapeutic "roads" that lead to recovery from mental health problems (Roth & Fonagy, 2005). No single approach can claim exclusivity or superiority in this respect, though if we directed our research efforts more productively to understanding the specificity of the different models for particular problems, we might get closer to identifying more reliable differences between modalities that actually do make a difference.

The social vertex

Alongside the developmental–relational vertices is the social vertex. In one sense the relational vertex is inherently about our social nature: we are social beings bound together, for better or worse, in intricate social networks. I am choosing to distinguish the social vertex from the relational one because if it is subsumed under the relational vertex, it may obfuscate the importance of social realities and processes and how these impact on mental health. For example, social exclusion, discrimination, and stigma still add to the suffering of people with mental health problems (and of those close to them). Fewer than a quarter of adults with long-term mental health problems are in work. They are nearly three times more likely to be in debt and can struggle for basic requirements of modern life like good housing or transport. Mental illness significantly increases the risk of unemployment, poverty, poor physical health, and substance misuse—and vice versa. There are persistent inequalities in mental health and in services, including those for black and minority ethnic communities.

The psychoanalytic emphasis on the internal world has often been criticized as being divorced from the social forces that also shape our individual experiences: our embodied existence in a world of social relations that unfold in a given socio-historical context. Here it could be argued that our systemic colleagues have managed more consistently to keep alive in their interventions the important interplay between the individual and his or her external context. But there is also a strong tradition of psychoanalytically informed thinking that emphasizes the social domain, and, importantly, some of it has developed from within this institution (e.g. Cooper & Lousada, 2005; Rustin, 1991). Indeed, the social dimension—strongly represented in this institution through an established tradition of social work practice and training, bearing the imprint of both psychoanalytic and systemic influences—is an essential voice reminding us that we are the products of our social and cultural environments. This voice has ensured that social care and mental health care remain connected—that there is a dialogue between them. If such dialogues are to make an actual difference, it is vital to go beyond the confines of this institution: we need to engage with policy makers, the media, and the users of our services.

The social perspective is also a potent reminder that the Tavistock and Portman Clinics are "social organizations" shaped by the same historical and contemporary cultural forces as the rest of society (Cooper & Lousada, 2005, 2010). They cannot exist outside this external context and need therefore to engage with it in a self-reflexive way.

The social vertex acts as an essential corrective to the belief that psychotherapy is sufficient to make a difference to people's lives. Although there is no doubt that enhancing the resilience of the individual or of a family increases the chance that they can engage with the external world with greater fortitude, it is also true that we live in an external word that is often beyond our individual control. In other words, psychotherapy per se (as separate from the set of ideas that underpin it and that may also be helpfully applied to an understanding of social processes) may be necessary, but it is not always—or even often—sufficient. Psychotherapy—irrespective of brand—only significantly helps, on average, around 50% of referred patients who complete their treatments (Fonagy, 2010; Westen & Bradley, 2005). This is not a bad outcome, but it is a sobering reminder that psychotherapy is not a panacea. A relationally based approach to mental health thus needs to be rooted in the broader sociocultural context in which our relationships are organized, because change is often also required at this level.

Thinking spaces

It is not only the patient who needs to be understood in his or her relational context. Several of the chapters in this book also speak to the importance of the relational context in which we work and how this impacts on our capacity to work.

The development of the work discussion model originated in the Tavistock Clinic. It embodies one of the distinctive values underpinning the work of this institution: the importance of thinking together. The psychoanalytically and systemically informed "work discussion" formats, respectively, as well as the systemic "reflective teams", underscore the acknowledgement that high-quality work with people with mental health problems requires a space for reflection both on the clinician's emotional reactions to the work with patients and on the experience of being part of an organization.

In approaching the work discussion format, some subscribe to the analytic view that the spotlight needs to be on unconscious, intersubjective mechanisms such as projection. Others find a more congenial home in the systemic view that it is narratives that determine how relationships unfold, and hence the focus needs to be on the relations between meanings that organize human relationships. These different positions nonetheless converge over the value of spaces where colleagues think about their work together.

Such spaces allow for the emotional experience of the work to be processed and for hypotheses to be shared so as to keep thinking alive. They support a process that, as a psychoanalyst, I would refer to as "learning from experience" (Bion, 1962)—that is, learning that is rooted in our emotional experience. This is a process that situates the so-called knower at the heart of the learning process. It is integral to the quality of what we offer because it can yield important information about the patient's state of mind and the functioning of a family, team, or organization. Our work engages at least two minds and, indeed, often several minds and subjectivities, and hence the risk of misunderstandings or enactments is considerable.

Such spaces also support a receptive state of mind in the practitioner, keeping alive conversations that might otherwise be closed down through "expertise and certainty" (Campbell & Groenbeck, 2006). Whichever model we subscribe to, such spaces enhance the resilience of the worker in the face of the sometimes violent and intrusive projections commonly encountered when working with particular patient groups (see chapter six, by Carine Minne, and chapter eight, by Jessica Yakeley).

Unfortunately, in the current NHS climate and under pressure to cut costs while increasing productivity, such thinking spaces have been all but eroded. They are seen as a "luxury" of bygone times that cannot be afforded. But this is a false economy: such thinking spaces are integral to what constitutes a quality service. A great deal of work has, in recent years, gone into developing competences for a range of psychological therapies (Roth & Pilling, 2008), but, if we really want to allow our patients to benefit from what psychological therapies have to offer, we have to address what makes for a competent service—that is, what support structures can sustain workers who are on the front line and are responding to high levels of psychic distress.

The container for our work—the organization in which we work— is a central aspect of the interventions we offer. Just as Winnicott (1960) drew attention to the crucial role of the father in supporting the evolving relationship between mother and baby, so, at its best, the organization we work in supports our work, providing and protecting the necessary conditions that allow us to devote our minds to the minds of our patients.

In practice this means that the organization—not just the one described here, but all organizations in this field of work—need to provide opportunities for reflecting not only on our direct work with patients, but also on the impact we have on each other as colleagues. Our need to take sides, to split, to be the favoured child, are revived and re-lived in our organizational lives. When we align ourselves to one group and not another, we are not solely driven by theoretical differences or scientific findings: we are also living out, for example, the fantasy that we have successfully relegated our rival to a less privileged group. Ideally, of course, the point of any kind of social organization should be to encourage the widest possible human diversity (Rorty, 1989, 1999), but anyone who has ever worked in a team will know that these dynamics are an inevitable part of group life.

In any organization we need not only internal spaces to talk with each other, but also fora to exchange ideas with colleagues working in other institutions and in other disciplines. By setting out our values, our work, and the challenges that we face, this book attempts to invite such an exchange beyond the boundary of our own organization.

Brave new worlds: good times, hard times, and beyond

In 1920, when Dr Crichton-Miller committed himself to helping the survivors of shell shock with psychotherapeutic interventions, he was engaged in innovative work. Since their inception, the Tavistock and Portman Clinics have facilitated the development of many original ideas and applications that have influenced generations of clinicians. But their heyday as bastions of psychoanalytic and systemic creativity can now seem far removed from the more mundane, and sometimes restrictive, present-day reality of service line reporting, payment-by-results, NICE guidelines, and evidence-based practice (EBP)—to name but a few of the drivers currently shaping health-care delivery and training in the United Kingdom.

The culture of EBP, though laudable in many respects, has also nevertheless had some unfortunate consequences for those therapeutic approaches that are not steeped in a scientist–practitioner model. Though I am a psychoanalyst, and this is sometimes thought to be incompatible with an interest in research, I welcome the current emphasis on EBP. It is also the case, however, that the sometimes not so nice NICE guidance has changed the commissioning landscape prioritizing certain approaches to the detriment of others. In many service contexts, the prioritization in this "highly politicized scientific environment" (Rustin, 2010), of cognitive behavioural therapy (CBT) on the grounds of its allegedly superior evidence base starkly highlights the precarious position of psychoanalytic and systemic therapies. And let us make no mistake about this: science may have its part to play, but this is also about politics. Scientific credentials do not provide immunity from the unconscious: within every scientist there is an individual fuelled by deep passions—just like the rest of us.

The *principle* of NICE guidelines is to be welcomed: it is incumbent on us as professionals to expose our work to scrutiny, so as to give those who use our services information about what we do and how effective we are. The demand to justify the effectiveness of what we offer provides a corrective against complacency. However, *how* the principle of accountability has been approached is another matter altogether. There are serious questions to be asked about the definitions of what constitutes "evidence", which are somewhat restrictive and privilege the randomized controlled trial as the gold standard of evidence, which is not without its limitations (Rawlins, 2008). This evidence hierarchy clearly disadvantages some therapeutic traditions that for a host of reasons have been slow, even reluctant, to engage in outcome research of this kind or at all (Fonagy, 2010).

It has not proven easy to rise to the challenge of EBP, not least because research is not embedded in the culture of most psychotherapy trainings (CBT being the exception). Many psychotherapists react with varying degrees of allergy to the requirement for outcome monitoring and to the manualization of the therapeutic encounter. Research is regarded as a rarefied activity, entirely divorced from the concerns of the clinician in the consulting room. The measures used to assess outcomes often seem to be irrelevant to what matters to patients. In this respect the recent governmental steer in the direction of "real" measures that matter to people's lives is welcome (DoH, 2010).

Of course, all knowledge is subject to both rational and irrational forces. It is vital to counter some of the more simplistic notions about the privileged status of scientific findings. Equally, however, if all knowledge is vulnerable to unconscious forces, this alerts us to the fact that our "clinical knowledge" is similarly compromised, so that, from whatever perspective we approach the task of understanding a phenomenon, we invariably need another perspective to act as a kind of corrective. Research can provide one such "other" perspective for the clinician, just as the clinician can alert the researcher to potential blind spots in his or her scientific field of vision. At its best, research can, and often does, support our clinical endeavours by providing a better understanding of our patients and of how we can help them through psychological interventions.

The future of mental health care in public health service contexts is uncertain. What is clear, however, is that the EBP agenda is here to stay. Engagement with this demand requires that we try out different ways of doing things, which may feel alien to established practice (such as session-by-session outcome monitoring) and to many may seem altogether irrelevant to what transpires in the therapeutic situation. Arguably this also requires that we actively respond to this external culture from a vantage point that is distinctively practice-based, so that we are not just "complying" with what we feel is imposed on us (although sometimes we have to do that too), but, rather, contribute to the discourse about varieties of scientific research and the contributions and limitations of different kinds of methodologies.

The uncertain future we face is also one of economic recession— the only certainty this offers up is that the money required to deliver high-quality services will always fall short of what is needed. How to survive without compromising the integrity of the values that underpin our interventions and of the models we espouse is the challenge we all face. Within this institution, this is a challenge that is being met with creative efforts that actively engage with the currency of the times, as is well illustrated, for example, by the developments in online therapeutic interventions (see chapter nine, by Richard Graham)—a far cry from the more controlled, physically tangible encounter in the consulting room. And if such developments may be felt by some to run counter to deeply held beliefs about what is helpful therapeutically, the voice of the user on these interventions is clear: they are felt to be helpful.

As several of the chapters in this book attest, the greater the complexity of the problems our patients present with, the greater the need to go beyond the confines of professional identities and theoretical allegiances. We also need to cross institutional boundaries to forge collaborations with other organizations (see chapter nine, by Richard Graham, and chapter ten, by Alessandra Lemma, Mary Target, & Peter Fonagy). This is true for many providers of psychological therapy services because we are all now competing for scarce resources. Collaborative efforts will become essential to survival and will require careful management of the process of "working together".

Collaborations across institutional divides can arouse suspicion and anxiety about being taken over by the "other". It may be difficult to integrate different traditions within one institution, but the challenge is all the greater when the actual and fantasized differences are concretely located in a separate institution, which stands for a foreign otherness that cannot be trusted. The threat of merger, of losing one's identity and core values, surfaces and risks undermining initiatives that have creative potential. Such cross-boundary initiatives can feel very destabilizing. Their management requires openness not only to what can be gained but also to what might be lost. This is one reason why collaborations require "work"; but their outcome is often a potent reminder that the whole is greater than the sum of its parts.

The way forward in mental health care—not only in this institution, but in any service that is in the business of helping people in psychic distress—requires us to be more integrative in our efforts.[5] By this I mean that we need to have more integrated, multi-model services, and we need to investigate the benefits of integrating different techniques/approaches where these might be more effective in helping particular patients. It might be a start if we could recognize where we are already doing this, even if we do not label it as such. We also need to integrate research more systematically into routine clinical practice. All this is easier said than done, as one patient reminded me. In response to an interpretation attempting to reconnect him with split-off aspects of himself, this insightful man wryly remarked: "Integration isn't all it's cracked up to be. Splitting keeps me sane!"

The merits of integration, as the patient observed, may well not feel as if they are what they are "cracked up to be". Integration requires painful psychic work. Klein describes the lifelong tension between the urge towards integration and the impossibility of sustaining a state of integration:

> Integration is difficult to accept. The coming together of destructive and loving impulses, and of the good and bad aspects of the object, arouses the anxiety that destructive feelings may overwhelm the loving feelings and endanger the good object. [Klein, 1963, pp. 301–302]

The challenge of integration is, for each of us, echoed in the process of engaging with an "other" experienced as a threat to our existence. The threat of disintegration mobilizes the urge to split off the disturbing otherness. This is especially pertinent to the perceived risks of collaboration with other institutions or ideas.

Greater "openness" to the reality of our incompleteness and, hence, our need for others (including other perspectives) exposes us to uncertainty—to internal and external forces that we can neither fully understand nor control. The "cure" for this uncertainty is often to retreat into certainties.

In engaging with what is essentially a more pluralistic mental health care context, the anxiety may be that as we take more in—into our minds and into our organizations—so the corporate body we feel identified with and comforted by will become a bit flabby around the core of our discipline, and the exercise of development will leave us uncertain about our readiness to compete. Whatever our group allegiances within the broader community of psychological therapies, we will all have to face a degree of survival anxiety in the current external climate. The only certainty we can have is that we will have to compete, and, sadly, we may not all be able to win and have prizes. This challenge is one that many services share beyond the boundary of this particular institution.

Extinction anxiety, whether real or imagined, raises the issue of adaptation in evolutionary terms. Evolution involves a changing response to a changing internal and external environment, and an uncertain adaptation is inherent in this process, which may involve the need for integration. This involves relinquishing a prior position that may nevertheless gradually enhance overall development.

As we face the challenges ahead in the related fields of mental health and social care, the best we can hope for from any organization that brings people together to relieve psychic pain is to create structures that authorize taking the time to reflect on the process of the work and how we relate to each other. This is the only way to support a sense of shared solidarity that is, in my view, an essential requirement for development. A sense of solidarity requires that we become far more self-reflective than our narcissism can probably bear to tolerate. Fundamentally, a sense of solidarity requires from all of us the ability to see in otherness the only things that truly unite us—namely, the potential for suffering and for hope, our need for beliefs, and our inevitable, often shared tendency to treat beliefs as if they were facts (Rorty, 1989).

In the face of external and internal pressures, the Tavistock and Portman NHS Foundation Trust continues to work hard to protect the importance of thinking spaces as integral to our clinical work and training activity. If it does not always manage to do this as well as we might like, its "good-enoughness" asserts itself in its continued willingness, at least, to try to think.

Notes

1. I shall refer to the Tavistock and Portman NHS Foundation Trust henceforth as the "Tavistock and Portman Clinics". When I refer to "the institution" or "the organization" I am referring to both Clinics, unless otherwise specified.

2. www.tavistockandportman.nhs.uk/aimstargets

3. Aristotle's "four causes theory" explains that the cause of "some thing" is based on the reason why this "some thing" is made.

4. The within-group differences about such matters are sometimes as great as, if not greater than, the apparent between-group differences.

5. This section is partly based on an Editorial I had the good fortune to co-write with James Johnston (Lemma & Johnston, 2010). I am grateful to him for his thoughts on the challenge of integration, some of which are included here.

References

Bion, W. R. (1962). *Learning from Experience*. London: Karnac, 1984.

Campbell, D., & Groenbeck, M. (2006). *Taking Positions in the Organization*. London: Karnac.

Cooper, A., & Lousada, J. (2005). *Borderline Welfare*. London: Karnac.

Cooper, A., & Lousada, J. (2010). The shock of the real: Psychoanalysis, modernity, survival. In: A. Lemma & M. Patrick (Eds.), *Off the Couch: Contemporary Psychoanalytic Applications*. London: Routledge.

DoH (2010). *Equity and Excellence: Liberating the NHS*. London: Department of Health/The Stationery Office. Available at: www.dh.gov.uk/health/search/?searchTerms=Liberating+the+NHS

Faimberg, H. (2005). *The Telescoping of Generations*. London: Routledge.

Fonagy, P. (2010). The changing shape of clinical practice: A comprehensive narrative review. *Psychoanalytic Psychotherapy*, 24 (1): 22–43.

Garland, C. (2002). *Understanding Trauma: A Psychoanalytic Approach*. London: Karnac.

Jenkins, R., Meltzer, H., Jones, P., Brugha, T., Bebbington, P., Farrell, M., et al. (2008). *Mental Capital and Wellbeing Project. Mental Health: Future Challenges*. London: Government Office for Science.

Kim-Cohen, J., Caspi, A., Moffitt, T., Harrington, H., Milne, B., & Poulton, R. (2003). Prior juvenile diagnoses in adults with mental disorder: Developmental follow-back of a prospective longitudinal cohort. *Archives of General Psychiatry*, 60: 709–717.

Klein, M. (1963). On the sense of loneliness. In: *Envy and Gratitude and Other Works* (pp. 300–313). London: Hogarth Press, 1975.

Lear, J. (2009). Technique and final cause in psychoanalysis: Four ways of looking at one moment. *International Journal of Psychoanalysis, 90*: 1299–1317.

Lemma, A. (2011). An order of pure decision: Growing up in a virtual world and the adolescent's experience of the body. *Journal of the American Psychoanalytic Association, 58* (4): 691–714.

Lemma, A., & Johnston, J. (2010). Editorial. *Psychoanalytic Psychotherapy, 24* (3): 179–182.

Rawlins, M. (2008). *De Testimonio: On the Evidence for Decisions about the Use of Therapeutic Interventions*. The Harveian Oration. London: Royal College of Physicians.

Rorty, R. (1989). *Contingency, Irony and Solidarity*. Cambridge: Cambridge University Press.

Rorty, R. (1999). *Philosophy and Social Hope*. London: Penguin.

Ross, W. D. (1950). *Physica*. Oxford: Clarendon Press.

Roth, A., & Fonagy, P. (2005). *What Works for Whom? A Critical Review of Psychotherapy Research* (2nd edition). New York: Guilford Press.

Roth, A., & Pilling, S. (2008). Using an evidence-based methodology to identify the competences required to deliver effective cognitive and behavioural therapy for depression and anxiety disorders. *Behavioural and Cognitive Psychotherapy, 36*: 129–147.

Rustin, M. (1991). *The Good Society and the Inner World: Psychoanalysis, Politics and Culture*. London: Verso.

Rustin, M. (2010). Varieties of psychoanalytic research. *Psychoanalytic Psychotherapy, 24* (4): 380–397.

Steiner, J. (1994). Foreword. In: J. Magagna (Ed.), *Universals of Psychoanalysis in the Treatment of Psychotic and Borderline Patients*. London: Free Association Books.

Westen, D., & Bradley, R. (2005). Empirically supported complexity: Rethinking evidence-based practice in psychotherapy. *Current Directions in Psychological Science, 14* (5): 266–271.

Winnicott, D. W. (1960). The theory of the parent–infant relationship. *International Journal of Psycho-Analysis, 41*: 585–595. Also in: *The Maturational Processes and the Facilitating Environment* (pp. 37–55). London: Karnac, 1990.

CHAPTER ONE

Talk talk:
theories and practices for turbulent times

Andrew Cooper

> Only by changing our institutional world can we change
> ourselves at the same time, as it is only through the desire to
> change ourselves that institutional change can occur.

David Harvey (2000, p. 186)

Mental health: hard labour

Stability or closure of our identities is an illusion. Too much change and transformation is intolerable. We seek closure as a refuge from the anxiety and mental turmoil it creates in us. We do this via the stories we tell about ourselves and others. These narratives structure our world, supported by and giving shape to powerful conscious and unconscious feeling states. But the stability of these emotional structures is illusory. They protect us at the same time as they limit our possibilities and freedom of thought and action. This is not a new paradox, but for individuals and organizations—especially those devoted to alleviating mental suffering—it is given fresh significance by the times. The political, intellectual, and policy culture we inhabit ceaselessly demands innovation, transformation, and renewal. Thus it promotes one side of the paradox and demotes the other, the necessity of illusions, the need for a place to rest and think.

Developed capitalist societies are traversing rapid and turbulent change following the economic crisis of 2008–09, and the theories, practices, and organizations that have for the last 50 years embodied their efforts to tackle social suffering, inequality, and mental pain in society are subject to radical questioning. In such times, some have argued that conservatism is a form of radicalism—the struggle to preserve progressive and humane social and organizational practices in the face of "modernization" becomes paramount. But how do mental health services draw a distinction between unhelpful resistance to change and the struggle to conserve a valuable and valued endeavour?

In this chapter I explore how the Tavistock tradition might help our understanding and handling of some of these contemporary dilemmas. These questions are not "just theoretical": emotional and social suffering is real, immediate, and damaging for those afflicted. The model of mind and social life sketched out in this chapter in answer to these questions is not simple, but arguably its validity has stood the test of time. It is not simple partly because, as the philosopher Jacques Derrida once said, "If things were simple, word would have gotten around". The paradoxes outlined above are part of the complexity, but they are often played out in an oppositional manner, as arguments involving entrenched positions taken by competing schools of thought and practice that could be supporting one another.

Historically, this is true within the Tavistock itself, and so this chapter attempts to model something that we all tend to preach but often find hard to practise—tolerance of difference, ambiguity, tension, or contradiction—in search of an integration of ideas. Broadly, this chapter suggests that each of the two main schools of therapy houses—family systems and psychoanalysis—tends to occupy a different side of the paradoxical coin, with psychoanalysis marginally favouring a narrative of stability and closure, and family systems one of openness and fluidity. But the difference between them may, on closer inspection, transpire to be credit-card thin, their argument with one another a case study in what Freud (1930a) called "The narcissism of minor differences". If this idea has validity, then it is transferable to many other instances of tension and conflict in contemporary organizational, social, and personal life.

Tavistock "philosophy" proposes that the best way to surmount entrenched states of hostility, conflict, intransigence, misunderstanding, or impasse is to put people in a room together and talk—anywhere between two and a hundred and two, as we shall see. Eventually, if things go well, some new version of the fixed, troublesome "truth" will emerge. This notion of knowledge or truth as a *process* of engagement, a dialogue leading to discovery, echoes the now rather unfashionable tradition of dialectical thought and philosophy. And, as the citations above suggest, I want to propose that this is also a helpful perspective for contemporary organizational life, as social institutions everywhere grapple with their identities in a period of turbulent change.

In common with many mental health service organizations, the Tavistock Clinic enterprise is a human project that tries to engage with some of the most profound, intractable, and painful realities facing us all. It is not "above and beyond" these realities but entangled with them and thus as vulnerable to their insidious and damaging aspects as are the people it tries to help. This chapter suggests that what unifies its different schools of therapy and practice is a commitment to direct engagement with lived human realities, in search of imaginative transformations that release people from incarcerating social and psychological pain and relationships. On this view, a potential for change and transformation is at the heart of what it means to be "mentally healthy"—but so, it turns out, is a capacity for stubbornness: "knowing your own mind" and what you stand for (and will not stand for), both personally and organizationally. The quest for that which "alters not when it alteration finds" is the heart of the matter. But in a period when change is visited on us by forces that seem beyond our control, the problem of how to navigate our personal and organizational identities *with integrity* becomes acute.

But if individuals and organizations dedicated to such helping practices are themselves subject to the same forces that act upon and within people seeking help, then the former must continually work to release themselves from the grip of self-incarceration, and this necessitates a dialectical movement between openness and closure. The tendency for psychotherapeutic practitioners and institutions to assume an omniscient and inferiorizing stance towards the suffering or afflicted "other" is evidence of the absence of such movement. The dedication of experienced mental health practitioners to continuing rigorous supervision and self-analysis signals its presence. The psychic and organizational strain of sustaining the continually self-questioning stance necessary for openness and transformation speaks to the contemporary requirement for "vulnerability" in our psychological stance as professionals (Hirschhorn, 1997) and the likely impossibility of sustaining a mental posture of perpetual "negative capability". Whatever you call it—reflexivity, self-awareness, deconstruction—staying "mentally healthy" is hard mental labour.

A bottom line?

The notion of an "enterprise" speaks to the fact that the work of the Tavistock, like most contemporary organizations, is not confined inside its geographically located organizational boundary (Cooper & Dartington, 2004). The enterprise is an "open system". It is the set of total exchange processes transacted among a wide range of cultural, professional, social, psychological, spatial, and temporal elements—the intersecting and overlapping relationships and movements among patients, trainees, professionals, public, the media—that constitutes the whole. Does this depiction reflect actual changes in organizational structure and form—a trend towards a more dispersed or networked form of organization with less well bounded spatio-temporal coordinates—or just a new way of seeing what has always been the case: a release from the *illusion* of well-bounded institutions with a clear, single primary task? Or maybe a complex blend of both in which new ways of seeing enable different ways of being and vice versa?

These questions haunt most modern organizations, as well as many key social institutions such as political parties. They also sound very like the questions people ask of psychotherapy itself—(how) can simple talk give rise to change, and have I really changed or just altered my view of myself, freed myself from constricting self-representations? However, there are important "realities" that are in tension with any view of organizations as somehow liberated from the straitjacket of tradition and modernity, free to impose themselves on the high seas of the market if only they have the self-belief to pursue a project of domination. The financial crisis of 2008–09 brought this home: money turns out not to grow on trees, even if temporarily it proved possible to persuade ourselves that it does. Ultimately the "bubble" burst because "sub-prime" home-owners from poor

American communities *could not pay* (Lanchester, 2010). It transpired that there is a "material" constraint on endless growth. Likewise, the Tavistock Centre building in Swiss Cottage, and other physical sites it now "owns", are obstinately there, housing expensive staff whose salaries consume most of the organization's budget, using heat and light that must be paid for. But by whom, why, and what for? If psychotherapy and organizational consultancy can make us a little freer, we should welcome this, but also not confuse freedom with immortality or omnipotence. Buildings crumble, water pipes burst, bodies age: we die or find that our credit has reached its limit, and no amount of "thinking it differently" can alter certain brute facts.

This chapter is about some of the invisible "technologies" that occupy the space between despair in the face of life's struggles and brute facts and the possibility of finding hope and meaning. They concern ways of engaging in personal, group, organizational, and social development evolved at the Tavistock over many decades, practised and refined every day by many thousands of people who have learned from them. These "methods" are directed at creating conditions for seeing and experiencing the self, relationships, and family and social relations in a different way. Thus, they are about liberating imaginative and imagined futures from the imprisoning hold that unconscious beliefs and emotions, languages and scripts, and restrictive or oppressive social and organizational practices can exert.

So, what are these "technologies"? After 90 years of Tavistock history, do they remain relevant to others in modern times? Are they evolving or static? Is there still hope for the vision of mind and social life they embody?

The observer

A child psychiatrist and family therapist who worked at the Tavistock Clinic for over 30 years was fond of saying: "You can observe the Tavistock's core technology any time you want to. Just walk down Fitzjohn's Avenue and look though the windows of the seminar rooms. What do you see? You see groups of people sitting in a circle, talking, thinking together."

He is right. But what are these people talking and thinking about? How can such a seemingly mundane and passive activity generate so much passion, commitment, and controversy? If there is anything in this method, can it be described, explained, made transparent, or is it a form of mystique as its critics and detractors often claim? Reviewing the first phase of a large consultancy intervention, I asked the CEO who had commissioned the intervention what the feedback was like. "Positive from a lot of people", he said. "And the others?" I asked. "In short, same old Tavi bollocks", he replied.

My approach to the writing of this chapter is deeply rooted in my own experience of working at the Tavistock as a teacher, clinician, manager, and consultant, but also as a learner and student. It is therefore necessarily personal, partial, and selective, but also questioning and critical. I have loved working and learning at the Tavistock. It has shaped my life in many respects. But this does not prevent me thinking, sometimes several times a day, "Aarrgh. . . . Same old Tavi bollocks."

The observer peering through the windows of the Tavistock is engaged in the very same "Tavistock" activity that so divides people's responses to this institution. He is looking, reflecting, wondering, formulating an idea and a concept for what he sees. He is thinking about an experience. Central to this is his awareness of his own mental processes which are focused on other people and what they might be up to. He is interested in "other minds" as well as his own. And so he is engaged in a relationship. Out of such simple but actually quite sophisticated mental activity is born the possibility of being a person with a mind, and of something called "society"—a system of relationships.

One, several, many, one . . . ?

There is not one single Tavistock model and method. As will become clear, both in this chapter and throughout the remainder of the book, there is in reality something more akin to an extended family constellation of ideas and practices, linked by a set of family resemblances. But how close is this family? Traditionally, the institution has thought of itself as housing two main clinical and theoretical paradigms—object relations psychoanalysis and systemic family therapy—although much of what the Tavistock is known for are extensions, ramifications, applications of these originating practices. In recent years, in response to shifting public and professional demands and forces in the mental health field, other clinical traditions, such as cognitive behavioural therapy, have found a foothold, and new models of short-term dynamic psychotherapy are being developed and tested. So far, it is unclear how this more inclusive trend will affect, or be affected by, the core methodological tradition. Change processes in individuals, couples, families, groups, and organizations are central to what the Tavistock Clinic and its services are all about, and as the wider world changes, so must the institution itself.

But how does change come about? And what makes up the more stable or perhaps "stuck" identity of the person or system of people that is endeavouring to change? Are there limits to the possibility of change, and if so, what are they? Investigating these questions will direct us to the heart of what Tavistock models and methods are about and reveal that although there is not a single or final answer, perhaps there is a deep structure, a relatively stable pattern, to the set of fundamental human predicaments—and ideas about these predicaments—with which the methods and models try to engage. Practitioners of psychoanalytic therapy and family systems therapy are more or less united on one thing: a certain kind of talk or conversation is essential to the possibility of change. This is why the people you can see through the windows of the seminar rooms could be teachers and learners within either tradition, or indeed both.

However, an investigation of the physical spaces within which Tavistock clinical practice occurs tells a different story. I once saw a family for assessment in the Adolescent Department psychoanalytic family therapy service. The young man who was the "index patient" walked into the room with his parents and immediately turned to me in alarm. "What's that?", he asked, pointing to one wall of the room. I think he half knew what it was. The wall was shuttered, and behind the shutter was a one-way screen. Beyond the screen was a second room, where, if this had been systemic family therapy, one or more clinicians—the reflecting team—would also have been sitting with the shutter open, so that they could observe the family while remaining invisible to that family. This scene can represent the point of departure for an important thread of the inquiry of this chapter. When we observe human behaviour and interaction as therapists, what are we attending to in our search to understand their pain and suffering? When we talk, what kinds of "insight" is our talk based upon? As clinicians, can we successfully observe ourselves without the help of others?

The two dominant traditions of psychotherapy at the heart of Tavistock practice transpire continually to divide, reunite, divide, and reunite around answers to these questions. This pattern of division and reunification may be the closest we can come to a "consensus" about Tavistock models and methods. The situation is perhaps analogous to that which faces theoretical physicists following the discovery of quantum mechanics. The deepest structure of physical reality seems to be a fluid and unpredictable contradiction, but it supports something—everyday physical reality—that appears stable and in many ways predictable. If comparison between the Tavistock tradition and the greatest achievements of modern science smacks of arrogance, perhaps this is a clue to the fiercely divided responses that the institution attracts, and also the continual emotional turbulence that is a feature of its daily working life. Adherents of the Tavistock's models and methods believe they really know something important. To others it can seem like dogma, a faith in obscure and arcane rituals that have little foundation in observable reality.

"Stop that fucking thinking!"

Whichever main tradition of practice and theory a person subscribes to, he or she might agree about one thing. The experience of being observed by others can feel intensely threatening. Perhaps this worry lay behind the reaction of the young man mentioned above on seeing the shuttered screen. I was introduced to this thought in my first hours of work at the Tavistock. I went to a meeting room and found two senior psychoanalysts there. I introduced myself, whereupon one of them declared, "It's a terribly difficult place to work, because everyone is scanning the unconscious the whole time!" "I'm not", responded her colleague. "Of course you are", said the first, "You must be. You're a psychoanalyst!" Whichever of these one takes to be nearer the norm, the presence of so many figures inside the institution who are *believed* to be scrutinizing each other may explain why, on entering the organization, perfectly well-balanced people often experience an acute discomfort that is also difficult to pinpoint.

Students on trainings who undertake planned observations of infants at home, or of organizational settings, frequently encounter unexpected resistance to the idea of "being observed". The reason is that the observer is often experienced as an intensely critical, judgemental presence rather than the interested, dispassionate one he or she believe him/herself to be. Being observed, and thought about, can feel very exposing—as though someone is "looking with x-ray eyes" into the murkiest and most shameful parts of the mind. Ronald Britton, a psychoanalyst who worked at the Tavistock for many years, has given much thought to the question of how and why some people come to be so terrified of their own minds that they cannot think about themselves, while others are much more at ease. He relates this to the nature of the relationship between the parental figures people carry inside themselves. If someone has a sense of parents who get together in a friendly way to think about them, then internal "mental space" can come to be established, a capacity to encompass feelings and thoughts about the self and others in a relatively free and easy way. But if the internal figures are felt to be too hostile or critical, ganging up against the child, then mental space closes down and the observing figures must be fought off. Britton describes working with a patient who, he believed, found his private efforts to "commune with himself" about her very threatening and burst out saying, "Stop that fucking thinking!" (Britton, 1989, p. 88).

Talk, experience, and "reality"

Psychoanalytic and systemic practice are united in questioning and interrogating the "surface" or taken-for-granted dimensions of how people represent themselves and their relationships in their talk. But they conceive of this project in somewhat different ways.

A psychoanalytic therapist had been seeing a woman twice weekly for a number of years. She found the patient consistently "difficult"—hostile, spiky, cryptic, unreflective—and often felt on the back foot, as though the patient was permanently at war with her, and winning. The patient often complained that the therapist wanted to impose her own theory or account of matters and did not take seriously the patient's own account of her troubles and their origins. Clearly, she did not feel "understood". The therapist acknowledged to herself and her supervisor that, unusually for her, she did not feel she easily recognized or identified with the patient. She felt her psychoanalytic work was rooted in many years of personal therapy, during which she had encountered in herself fragments or vestiges of most states of mind her patients presented to her. But this woman had always seemed different, and the therapist often felt she was failing the patient.

One of the patient's complaints was that the therapist wilfully ignored her belief that her emotionally isolated childhood had been blighted by "lack of social contacts", an absence of friendships. The therapist did indeed consistently probe other ways of understanding the patient's childhood—and adult—isolation. But these efforts always resulted in a "rupture" between the therapeutic couple. Then one night, after several years of this work, the therapist had a dream involving the patient. She described it as the most lucid dream she had ever had about her analytic work. In the dream, *she returned to her childhood home for a weekend to meet some friends and go for a walk. But she had also invited the patient to accompany her. On arriving at the house, she became worried about leaving the patient alone there while she met her friends and wondered whether she should not forgo the walk and keep her patient company. This is what she did, after rendezvousing with her friends and explaining.* The dream prompted the therapist to remember how isolated her own childhood had been in many ways, and how anxiously attached to her own mother she remembered becoming. On one occasion, the therapist's mother had gone away for the day and arranged for her daughter to travel by herself to visit a favourite aunt. But the young therapist had been frightened, feigned illness, and stayed at home with her father.

The therapist spoke of this experience in psychoanalytically familiar terms: she described how, in the dream, the patient was clearly "a part of herself"—the anxious, isolated child she thought she had long ago left behind. Her decision to stay at home and keep company with the patient, forgoing the pleasures of "social contact", both echoed the patient's talk of her own childhood and reminded the therapist of how anxious she herself had once been. Much to her surprise, since she believed herself to be a "well-analysed" therapist and fully conscious of her own childhood loneliness, she now believed that she had long been in a defended state with respect to this patient's own painfully withdrawn and isolated experiences.

Perhaps this vignette crystallizes something of how psychoanalysis "thinks"; it may help to explain how psychoanalytic work is done, as well as why it can feel so threatening. In psychoanalysis there is always a quest to look within or beyond a representation—in words or images—for signs of other representations, layers of psychic "reality" that infuse one another with meaning and feeling. The assumption is that these representational layers connect with one another, although not necessarily in a fixed or permanent way. Indeed, psychoanalytic work may be dedicated to revealing such connections in order to allow them to de-couple. Fixed, layered ways of thinking and feeling about the self and relationships may be at the root of the mental pain or symptomatology that first brings a person, family, or couple to therapy. Once disclosed, the faculties of the conscious mind can observe these layers of connectedness and re-assess them. This is a way of restating some of Freud's original formulations about psychoanalysis and how our minds work. "Free association" was the means of revealing the unexpected but meaningful series of connections, and the concept of the "primary process" contained his account of the "laws" of unconscious thought processes that generate them.

But how do we know whether this account is right? What justifies the assumption that different representational layers of thinking and experience connect in a particular way? Are there not deep and unexamined assumptions at work here about what lies "beyond" or "behind" manifest experience or surface talk, whether of dreams or other registers of experience. In fact, the therapist's assumption that "the patient stands for a part of herself" in the dream is a deeply "theory-laden" proposition. Her "story" about the dream is just that—a story—and, moreover, exactly the kind of story that a psychoanalytic therapist would tell under such circumstances, because the stories they tell are scripted according to assumptions of just this sort.

Suddenly it looks as though psychoanalysis can be hoisted on its own petard, its own discourses vulnerable to the same unexamined and fixed beliefs about how things are connected that it purports to be so good at disclosing in the thinking of others. Moreover, experience would suggest that were the therapist to narrate the dream a second time, the narrative would be subtly different and probably suggestive of new or differently nuanced interpretations or thinking. Or, because they usually cannot resist doing so, other psychoanalytic therapists hearing or reading this "story" will want to add, "But it could also mean. . . ." Which is the "true" or valid narration, and where do we find access to any core or "real meaning", as distinct from its various possible narrations? If there is a "reality" beyond the range of stories we can tell about an experience, access to it seems to be denied by the slipperiness of the same portal—language—that promises us entry to "the real". Under these circumstances, philosophical integrity surely demands that we focus attention on what can be more certainly grasped—namely, how people talk, narrate, tell stories about themselves and their relationships.

Once this shift of focus has been achieved, questions about whether there is or is not anything "beyond" talk that need concern us may just dissipate. Perhaps there is such a realm, but what we can now assert is that experience, relationships, states of mind—everything that is the proper object of a concerned therapist or mental health professional—is "constructed" through language and story-telling. If painful and disabling states of mind or relationship can be produced in this way, they can also be "deconstructed" through therapeutic work that encourages us not just to "tell it like it is" but to "tell it differently". Transformational conversations rather than a search for "truth" become the watchword.

Narratives of difference, similarity, resemblance . . .

Given these areas of convergence and divergence, how similarly or differently do therapists of different persuasion actually work and conceptualize such work? And do the practices themselves provide further clues to the nature of the elusive unity-in-diversity of the Tavistock's models? These are large questions, explored more fully in other parts of this book. Here I will confine myself to one important dimension of the answer that may signal a further "conjunction of differences". Both schools of therapy are committed to a view that the work cannot be done without a live, here-and-now, self-conscious entanglement of the therapist in the process of the work. Systemic therapists call this reflexivity, and psychoanalytic practitioners call it working with the transference and countertransference. Each entails its own idea of self-observation.

When a family or couple meets the systemic therapist(s), who, classically, will be supported by the presence of a reflecting team or colleague, the meeting is conceived as a joining of one system to another. This joining occurs through the medium of communication—not only talk but also other visible and describable communications: who sits where in the room, who opens the narration, who supports the terms of the dominant narrative, who might be dissenting from it through silence, and so on. The therapists, in turn, are invited to "join" this communicative pattern in particular ways and not to disrupt or question it in others. Their contributions cannot but confirm or disconfirm particular patterns or scripts. There is no "neutral" communicative stance, only an evolving co-production of new here-and-now patterns that will reinforce certain constructs in the "client system" and/or disturb and perhaps re-frame others.

Somewhere in this web of communicative patterns and silences, or told and untold story lines, lie the sources of, and possible solutions to, whatever difficulties have brought the system to therapy. As the therapists become "positioned" within the developing conversation, their observing faculty—themselves positioned out of sight behind the screen, but in contact with the process—may intervene to propose adjustments to the therapists' conversational strategies with respect to those of the family. This is talk about talk about talk, and the account you are reading is talk about talk about talk about talk; if you were now to discuss this with your friend, then it would be talk about talk about talk about talk about talk.

Part of the aim of therapeutic intervention in this modality of work might be to encourage the articulation of previously unheard or unvoiced "lines of narrative". The children may never have heard the parents speak of their own childhood difficulties; the parents may never have heard a child's account of their experience of the parents' arguments; everyone may have been silent since mother's miscarriage or father's redundancy. In systemic therapy a central aim is to keep the narratives moving, developing, shifting, open. As this process unfolds, an observing psychoanalytic therapist would be engaged by, and interested in, aspects of the total experience that the systems therapists seem to focus on less. For example, if a parent immediately engages one of the therapists, or one of the children, in a critical and disparaging manner, the interest is likely to focus on the powerful feelings involved in the exchange and what this may mean in terms of projective processes within the family. If the therapist suddenly feels small, useless, and unable to speak for fear of provoking another attack or creating an argument, she may speculate that this provides insight into how anxieties associated with dependency or insecurity are managed in the family. People are not just silenced from talk about such matters by particular communicative strategies, they are also made to feel small and stupid by those who find these very subjective states too hard to bear for themselves. Feeling like this can be very close to believing it to be true. In this way, the structure or patterning of the "system" becomes deeply inscribed in individual subjectivities as well as residing in interpersonal relationships that continually reinforce and reproduce these more private states of mind.

From here the psychoanalytic inquiry may begin to follow lines similar to those outlined above with respect to the therapist's dream. What deeply inscribed emotional experience and beliefs about being a child does the parent import into this family from his or her own experience of being parented? In other words, what is the *internal* grandparental and great grandparental "system" inhabiting this family in the here-and-now? Disclosing the continuing presence and influence of these absent or long dead figures, the family ghosts, may become an important focus of therapy. Enabling family members to speak of these formative experiences and memories constitutes psychoanalytic story-telling.

Feet on the ground or head in the clouds? Reflexivity and countertransference

As the psychoanalytic therapist consults herself about her own immediate experience of feeling attacked and disparaged, she tries to sort out its meaning. Is this a communication, via projection, of how a child typically comes to feel in this family when the parent reacts to feeling threatened? Is it how the parent experiences his or her own internal parental figures? Is it about the contemporary anxiety of starting therapy? Is the therapist herself especially sensitive to critical attacks of this kind? Or maybe all of these?

In systemic theory and practice there is, as we have seen, a trend towards the interminable re-framing of narratives via meta-perspectives on each narrative layer. In psychoanalytic thinking, there is an equivalent trend towards infinity in the search for both lateral and biographical associations of meaning and feeling. On the face of it, one appears to direct attention outwards and one inwards, the former linking systemic theory to the work of holistic philosophers like Gregory Bateson and Spinoza and the latter to traditions of mysticism, an association explicitly invoked by one of the most prominent psychoanalytic ghosts walking the corridors of the Tavistock—Wilfred Bion. Reflexivity can be described as the discipline of thinking about thinking and talking about talk so as to constantly interrogate and locate one's own position within a system; attention to the counter-transference is the discipline of continually scrutinizing the subjective states aroused in the therapist in order to locate evidence for one's position within the field of unconscious mental activity generated by the therapy. Both are central to the working practices of the Tavistock, and both signal an important paradox or tension about the institution's position within the contemporary cultural and social field.

Does the centre hold?

So, does a therapist of either—or, indeed, any—persuasion occupy a privileged position with respect to her *knowledge* of the individuals, families, or organizations she encounter and tries to work with? I have represented both systemic and psychoanalytic practice as constituted by a kind of radical scepticism, and yet the institution of the Tavistock is often portrayed as a centre of dogmatism. We live in an everyday world increasingly defined by professed ideologies of choice and relativism, a "post-traditional" and "post-hierarchical" world in which "difference" and multiplicity of perspective replace unity and dependence on received authority—sometimes as descriptions of how things *are*, sometimes of how they *should* be, or of both. Psychoanalytic and systemic thought have played a part in bringing this world into being. In different ways, both have contributed to "de-centring" the knowing subject from a privileged position with respect to itself and others. The necessary immersion or entanglement of the therapist with the psychic and systemic life of the "patient", and the correlative need to be permanently engaged in freeing or locating oneself, is one index of this.

Yet both schools would wish to defend their respective contributions to modern mental health work as solid, even necessary, to the possibility of good practice. People who come to the Tavistock to learn often say that they quickly feel themselves to be better grounded, more confident of their own position in relation to the intense emotional and intellectual complexities of their work. On the other hand, at the heart of the "Tavistock bollocks" lobby's complaint is a frustration with a perceived reluctance to just get "stuck in" rather than engage in ceaseless reflection. To ask that we reconcile these positions might be to fall prey to the very desire for unity and cohesion; the search for a master narrative that I have suggested is antithetical to the spirit of Tavistock thought. Is this the final paradox? Perhaps, perhaps not. . . .

A method for the madness

How do these various interlocking principles of therapy translate to the domain of teaching and learning? Writing about the practice of "Work Discussion", one of the central pedagogic Tavistock methods, Sebastian Kraemer says:

> There is an atmosphere of candour, even of risk, in which it is possible to say things that feel prejudiced or "judgemental". This is not a license to offend, but to speak from the heart . . . every discussant is regarded by the facilitator as presenting different *but equally valid* aspects of the case or theme.[1]

Again, we notice the theme of "participatory democracy", now threaded through the therapeutic learning process. In her discussion of this method, Margaret Rustin writes that:

> The aim is to strive for a relatively theory-free and non-judgemental attitude to everyone involved, including oneself. The apparently meaningless is just as valuable in the record as the probably or obviously significant. The debt to the free association method in psychoanalysis is an obvious one. [Rustin, 2008, p. 11]

The approach is also much informed by Bion's concept of "containment" or "container/contained", perhaps *the* most revered (and important) of psychoanalytic ideas in Tavistock discourse.

Given much of what has been said in the preceding pages, it might seem that we could characterize the entire Tavistock project as one of "containment": an institutional effort to create conditions in which "unthinkable" experiences in the minds and relationships of patients, professionals, organizations, and citizens can be rendered "thinkable" and speakable. In the psychoanalytic paradigm, the struggle is towards representability and language. In the systemic, it is rather more with the representations and forms of speech or language we already have.

Inability to represent and verbalize emotional experience can be disabling, imprisoning, a form of traumatic mutism; the discourses we do create are sometimes liberating, sometimes constraining and/or oppressive, and often both. Discourse *is* closure, and closure generally excludes or "others" one or another group or individual. The *experience* of authentically "free-associative" psychoanalytic work is that you never tell it the same twice over. Instability of "representation" is the norm. A fundamental precept of systemic work is that this is how it ought to be, if conditions for growth, change, development, and the realization of transformational possibilities are to be sustained. Psychoanalysis is good at showing us how unconscious processes and defences—splitting and projection—generate closed or compartmentalized psychic structures and systems. Systems thinking is good at disclosing the discursive strategies and formations that constitute the (micro-, meso-, macro-) social embodiment of these. Spaces of hope, rather than of despair, are dependent upon the contributions of both to producing cultures of liquidity.

The start of the world

Is there a Tavistock practice where these world views meet and exchange notes? The answer is perhaps yes and no. The tradition of group relations work *should* be a main site of rapprochement and is perhaps becoming so. The tension concerns how psychoanalytic and systems practitioners understand "systems" and work with them. The latter tend perhaps to see the former as having appropriated their systemic territory in a naïve psychoanalytic manner, while the former find the tendency of the latter to ignore "unconscious process" difficult. Nevertheless, alongside work discussion, group relations events are probably the most original Tavistock contribution to the study of "ordinary madness". Lasting anywhere between 3 and 14 days, with between 25 and 100 members, the central learning task of these events is to "study" the experience and process of the various small and large groups that constitute the whole "temporary institution". Group relations events bring into being a small, complex society, a full-blown "psychodynamic system".

To be part of the first minutes of a group relations event is rather like being present at the origin of the universe itself, or the birth of a child. First nothing, then something, and then awareness of this something; finally, perhaps, a name for it is spoken. But this can be harder than it sounds. At the start of one such conference, the hundred or so members were invited to gather in the large room available for "whole-system events", together with the conference staff, a number of whom positioned themselves at the edges of the space. The task was to form into groups of eight and select a member of staff as facilitator, thus forming the "small study groups" that would meet throughout the life of the conference. No guidance was offered about *how* to achieve this objective, except that it must be done in silence.

As people circulate silently around the room, small knots begin to form: pairs, threes, fours. They know they must eventually coagulate into groups of eight. A group of four meets one of three, and they decide to join. Lacking a final member, they look about themselves. Small groups that have not become attached search for possible partners. In less than half a minute, only a very few individuals have not attached themselves to someone else. Groups of nine or ten are now obliged to negotiate silently about who might leave them and search for another home. The first groups of eight begin to "dock" with group leaders positioned at the edges of the room. Somehow, after a few minutes, a dozen groups of eight people and twelve group leaders are linked to one other. They begin to leave the room to begin the first of their small study group sessions.

Taking up the task of the conference, one small group begins to reflect upon the experience of its own formation. Members speak about the anxiety, terror even, of finding themselves isolated and homeless. Some pairs and threes describe how they had instantaneously clung to one another on the basis of prior familiarity. Others say that all other members of the small group are unknown to them.

The group starts to reflect upon the mysterious process by which they selected their leader, and one member says that she tried to guide the group towards him because "he looked friendly", which perhaps signals the depth of the underlying fears already aroused. The group leader, in his turn, is thinking about what he is hearing, as well as his own experience of group formation. After a few minutes he intervenes and says that two thoughts occur to him to help make sense of this: "survival" and "any port in a storm. . . ."

These events are the experiential counterparts of philosophical ideas developed within other traditions, recalling, for example, Martin Heidegger's existentialist notion that each of us is "thrown" into the world and struggles ever after to live authentically with the terror of this condition, which is not of our choosing. The scientist and philosopher Jesper Hoffmeyer starts his book *Signs of Meaning in the Universe* (1996) by speculating about the evidence for material ripples or "scar tissue" left over from the big bang when the first "lumps in the universe" formed, producing the differentiation that is the necessary precondition of meaning and, eventually, communication.

The opening phases of the above conference replicate this chaotic, turbulent process of something—human groups—forming irrevocably out of the homogeneous soup of the totality. But they also speak to the unconscious terrors that lurk beneath the everyday ebb and flow of organizational and social life, the intimacy of strangers, the fear of abandonment and isolation, the ubiquitous propensity for intergroup rivalry, hatred, and cooperation.

An alternative space: the Democratic Republic of Swiss Cottage

So, do not be seduced or persuaded by the apparent calm, the *very thoughtful* atmosphere you might detect as you peer through the windows on Fitzjohn's Avenue. This is just an important outward display masking an equally important inner turbulence and turmoil. At their point of contact, as we have seen, is talk, language, and some other processes that inform talk both from "within" and from "without" in order—this is the hope—to generate meaning, understanding, and change.

In order to enter the main building of the Tavistock, you are obliged to step through a glass doorway, turn right for a few paces, go through another glass door, and then turn left. This peculiar arrangement has survived a recent refurbishment of the whole entrance lobby. Occasionally one can observe perplexed first-time visitors to the building twisting and turning as they try to fathom the way through. It is hard to think of another modern public building with a more convoluted boundary-crossing point. On the other hand, the Tavistock is one of the least "securitized" of public spaces—no passes, no signing in and out, not much CCTV. All day, from 7:30 in the morning until well past 9:00 in the evening, there is a constant flow of people in and out, sidestepping one another in the glass of the entrance—staff, patients, students, visiting teachers, guests, conference participants. Unless you are very familiar with the day-to-day activity of the institution, it is nearly impossible to identify who among these people belongs to which group, and in different ways a high proportion can lay claim to several of these identities.

The corridors of the clinical directorates in the building suggest a different story. Sequestered, noiseless (the rooms are excellently sound-proofed), anonymous except for tiny brass nameplates, the lines of uniform brown wooden doors are normally closed. An occasional one may reveal an open-plan office space, but more typically they house the clinical, teaching, managerial, and administrative staff, with many rooms trebling up as office and clinical and teaching space. At first sight it seems anyone can stroll into the Tavistock and wander through its mostly uniform spaces, as though it were an oversized, misplaced public library or art gallery—there are modern paintings hanging in almost every available wall space. But from time to time you will catch sight of two or more people making their way towards one of the offices silently, awkwardly—therapist and patient, or maybe family or group, arriving for (psychoanalytic) therapy. What happens between them behind the closed door, in the sound-proofed room, is intensely private and strictly "out of bounds" to anyone else. You can gain easy access to the Tavistock for many purposes, but, equally, many of its core activities and spaces are tightly patrolled. The position of the sliding vacant/engaged sign on each door is a key signifier of the continually oscillating transitional space between openness and closure, private and public, inner and outer worlds, that the Tavistock exists to study and engage with.

The creative tension—and synergy—between the necessarily privatized space of the therapeutic and the location of the Tavistock within the NHS and public sector was for many decades embodied in its unique internal structure of management and decision making: hierarchical, tribal, paternalist on the one hand; democratic, fluid, complex, and subversive on the other. Until the system was abolished in 2005 by the Board of the newly formed "Foundation Trust", the clinical staff of the organization elected all its own managers for fixed-term periods of office. These practices were understood as extensions of the models of mind and psychotherapy found at work behind the closed doors of the many corridors. Therapy is a process of helping people to recover agency and *authority* for the living of their own lives. Authority of any kind cannot be simply claimed or asserted or "supposed"; it must be found, discovered, conferred. Within a group it must be *both* granted and accepted or "taken up". This kind of democracy and authority is both elective and also—continually—participatory, because leaders and followers are in permanent relationship with each other.

But, once again, do not be seduced, however admirable, appealing, and progressive this model of organizational life may seem. Under the surface of democratic "maturity" and sophisticated notions of authority, naked urges for power and domination continue to lurk. In recent years, more than one medical consultant has been heard to voice the idea that doctors are in truth *primus inter pares* (first among equals) among the professions, thereby doubly enraging colleagues with an assertion of superiority cloaked in arcane language. Some exponents of some Tavistock clinical orientations have subtly abandoned courtesy and "participation" in favour of arrogant stances towards patients and students. Perhaps all clinical groupings and many individuals are guilty of such regressive behaviour at least some of the time. But each instance that affects a patient, student, or member of the community damages the Tavistock, providing ammunition for those who wish to attack its reputation and self-idealizations.

But for many the strong conviction persists that the loss of this 75-year-long tradition of therapeutic republicanism may have marked a decisive shift in the Tavistock's fortunes in the modern world. The boardroom battle that decided its fate was nasty, brutish, and short. Within the managerialist climate of the modern NHS, under the scrutiny of the ominously titled "Monitor" who oversees the governance and performance of Foundation Trusts, it was almost certainly unrealistic to hope that a democratic model of management could survive. Better, then, to kill it first, rather than face its extermination by an outside force? These are the decisions any "organizational ego" must confront in assessing its relationship to "external realities".

Democracy is one of the organizing principles of all "therapeutic communities", a tradition of residential "milieu" psychotherapy, with which the work of the Tavistock has much in common. Therapeutic provision of this kind has had a difficult time in the NHS in recent years and may be dying out within the British public sector. Therapeutic democracy is subversive, challenging the norms and practices of mainstream psychiatry and mental health practice, research, theory, and ideology. Uneasily positioned within mainstream NHS structures and its modern instruments of "governance", and so often seen by those who do not know or understand its practices as a centre of traditional elitism, the Tavistock's claim to radical status is often disputed. To those who do know it and have worked or learned there, its claim to represent a true alternative is not much in question. In a period of managerialist conformity, however, its capacity for long-term survival as a true "Other" is facing new challenges.

Through the decades, the Tavistock has negotiated many challenges to its future. If such challenges ceased, this would surely signal that it had already lost its institutional potency. Its core purpose is to disturb "the order of things" and of language, in pursuit of such freedom from everyday personal and social suffering as can be attained. Perhaps this is the lot of all organizations dedicated to improving mental health. Our society is deeply ambivalent about the mental pain it causes people and suffers in return and responds with equal ambivalence to those institutions that aim to engage and work with this pain. Tavistock theories and methods offer some hope that all of this turbulence can be made at least "thinkable" and thereby rendered a bit less toxic and destructive.

We can never "bound free" once and for all from the unconscious, language, or society, so the project is a never-ending struggle. We cannot live without "closures", but every settled state, equilibrium, unexamined assumption, or habit of organizational mind that helps constitute the creative "authority" of an institution is also the basis for possible corruption, oppression, and ultimately death. An organization whose purpose is transformational must be prepared for, and capable of, self-transformation.

Note

1. From a draft of an unpublished paper, "The Dangers of This Atmosphere: A Quaker Connection in the Tavistock Clinic's Development", written in 2009. A revised version was later published in the journal *History of the Human Sciences* (Kraemer, 2011).

References

Britton R. (1989). The missing link: Parental sexuality in the Oedipus complex. In: R. Britton, M. Feldman, & E. O'Shaughnessy, *The Oedipus Complex Today: Clinical Implications* (pp. 83–101). London: Karnac.

Cooper, A., & Dartington, T. (2004). The vanishing organization: Organizational containment in a networked world. In: C. Huffington, D. Armstrong, W. Halton, L. Hoyle, & J. Pooley (Eds.), *Working below the Surface: The Emotional Life of Contemporary Organizations* (pp. 127–150). London: Karnac.

Freud, S. (1930a). *Civilization and Its Discontents. Standard Edition*, 21.

Harvey, D. (2000). *Spaces of Hope*. Edinburgh: Edinburgh University Press.

Hirschhorn, L. (1997). *Reworking Authority: Leading and Following in the Post-Modern Age*. Cambridge, MA: MIT Press.

Hoffmeyer, J. (1996). *Signs of Meaning in the Universe*. Bloomington, IN: Indiana University Press.

Kraemer, S. (2011). The dangers of this atmosphere: A Quaker connection in the Tavistock Clinic's development. *History of the Human Sciences*, 24 (2): 82-102 .

Lanchester, J. (2010). *Whoops! Why Everyone Owes Everyone and No One Can Pay*. London: Penguin, Allen Lane.

Rustin, M. (2008). Work discussion: Some historical and theoretical observations. In: M. Rustin & J. Bradley (Eds.), *Work Discussion: Learning from Reflective Practice with Children and Families* (pp. 3–21). London: Karnac.

CHAPTER TWO

A plurality of just answers

Bernadette Wren & Ellie Kavner

Multiple identities and tribal loyalties

With the introduction of a more competitive, outcomes-oriented, and micro-managed NHS political economy, many mental heath institutions have become ideological battlefields where struggles for disciplinary primacy are being waged daily. In our workplace, rival modalities—articulating competing theories about and remedies for troubled behaviour relationships and inner worlds—are often seriously out of sympathy with each other. Many staff express anxiety about the way one model may gain favour over another within the NHS, and a fierce determination to defend time-honoured principles and practices in their clinical and teaching work.

With backgrounds in clinical psychology (BW) and social work (EK), we are two systemic psychotherapists working in an NHS institution, the Tavistock and Portman Trust, facing a future full of uncertainty. How and where we will be working in another five or ten years' time is unpredictable. But, whatever is to come, we think there are a number of related risks attached to our adherence to the often sharp boundary marking that informs the working practices in our own and other mental health services.

In our work we are both engaged in multiple roles in training, clinical practice, management, and research. Like many colleagues, we think we avoid being rigid in the reach of our ideas. We engage regularly with discourses from systems theory, sociology, developmental psychology, psychoanalysis, philosophy, politics, and social learning theory. Our work as managers and clinicians is often cross-disciplinary, and we enjoy our cross-modal interchanges. We are aware that many of the names most proudly associated with our institution drew on ideas and insights from a range of disciplines to develop powerful and influential new models of explanation and intervention.

Indeed, on the face of it, numerous disciplinary identities are available for people working in clinical, research, and teaching posts in mental health. One's professional self may be linked to one's original profession, one's psychotherapy training of choice, the client group with whom one has developed some expertise, and the setting of the work. In our Trust the development of services in community settings, once thought highly unlikely places for psychotherapies to thrive, with people who might once have seemed unlikely candidates for therapy, has necessitated a high degree of flexibility and adaptability in the choice of modes of intervention. The context of such work—schools, special-needs teams, GP practices, baby clinics, community drop-in centres—can press for the convergence of ideas about what approaches are required and possible.

But such seemingly multiple opportunities to build a layered professional identity often belie the extent to which many people experience the world of mental health as rigidly organized, permitting little interplay between different ideas and approaches. Practitioners, allied with others in their professional discipline and/or their therapeutic modality, often set great store on emphasizing differences in their precepts and praxis. The virtues of cross-modal working may be trumpeted at an institutional level, but attempts at collaboration frequently falter: innovative cross-disciplinarity seems elusive. In scholarly work, cross-citation between modalities is rare. Like many, we experience the strong tug of tribal loyalty when our guiding principles are misunderstood or undervalued and a sense of pleasure in cleaving to our preferred disciplinary or modality-based certainties. But our failures in this regard remain local and personal and do not often become occasions for institutional self-examination.

In this chapter we reflect on what we have learned about why it can be so difficult to work together among differences and how we might respond from an organizational point of view to the challenge to support cross-disciplinary and multi-modal work. We consider what would help people to function with more generosity and curiosity towards their colleagues from different modalities. In doing so, we explore the dangers of ossification, the fear of losing creative energy, and the obstacles to renewal.

Disciplinary responses to changing contexts

The new political economy of the NHS has come to embrace the apparatus of evaluation and controlled outcome research, the presentation and debate of results, and a range of techniques for the micro-assessment of practitioners. While it is widely argued that the primacy of evidence in medicine—designed to ensure that money is allocated efficiently and that patients are protected through knowledge of the most effective treatments—has translated awkwardly into the world of mental health, services have been obliged to make a commitment to routine assessment and outcome monitoring and to learning ways to promote, evaluate, and sell their services. The idea that science will determine how people can be helped has gained strength. Psychotherapeutic models that show their quality through good randomized controlled trials (RCTs) deserve to do well, it is argued, and should push others out of the marketplace. The NHS, we are told, should not support unproven psychotherapies, no matter how well-meaning and well-liked. Unsurprisingly, treatments that ostensibly make a better fit with the technologies of standardized assessment are those like cognitive behavioural therapy and structured parenting group work whose methods are largely rational and based on the client establishing treatment goals, learning new skills, and testing out beliefs.

Alongside these changes have also been moves, welcomed by many, for the greater involvement of patients/clients in their services. The expressed wishes of clients are increasingly accorded respect, options for treatment are outlined to them, and their views on their experience of therapy are sought. These various transformations have created a new context for considering how well the established psychotherapy schools are serving the public and whether further innovation, determined collaboration, or a return to tradition is most needed.

For the Tavistock and Portman, these changes within the NHS have been dramatic. Until the introduction of the internal market in the 1990s, the institution thrived for several decades within a mostly benign and stable NHS context, staff working almost exclusively in psychodynamically informed ways, with family systems psychotherapy developing in the Child and Family Department in the 1970s a small but active clinical team.[1] The last ten years have seen the introduction of a range of brief therapies—such as structured interpersonal therapies, parent training, and cognitive behavioural therapy. While some staff see these as psychologically naive interventions whose effectiveness has been greatly exaggerated, others see this widening of brief and pragmatic treatment options as a progressive change forced on an essentially conservative and elitist institution.

Reading of the Tavistock and Portman's history suggests that innovation in the face of changing times is nothing new, that adapting models to novel settings and client groups is an activity that has long been a recognizable part of the Tavistock and Portman's intellectual and operational repertoire. In Dicks' history of the institution published in 1970, he clearly demonstrates that in its early days the Tavistock pioneered an approach that was avowedly eclectic and multidisciplinary:

> While psychodynamic, the Clinic's doctrine beyond this general orientation was to "have no doctrine", but only aims: to help, to understand more and to teach its work. As such it was the meeting-ground of psychotherapists of several schools or of none, making for a certain vagueness and lack of theoretical homogeneity, but also for flexibility and a wide variety of techniques and viewpoints. [Dicks, 1970, p. 2]

While Dicks allows for doctrine-free thinking only within the confines of a broadly psychodynamic thought-space, his perspective on theoretical heterogeneity is, nevertheless, striking. The current crisis tends in contrast to evoke feelings of intense anxiety about the capacity of institutions to meet the challenge of change without catastrophic loss of core ways of working and teaching. Patrick writes about reactions to the way psychoanalysis in the public sector has evolved:

> We can come to feel that even evolution involves an abandonment of our internal objects. So electrically charged is the history of

psychoanalysis that such crimes can feel quite unforgivable. . . . Our household gods, and indeed our cultural superegos are powerful entities. [Patrick, 2010, p. 9]

This kind of anger and fear in response to change may be presented simply as a passionate concern to defend a venerable and valued model of clinical and teaching practice. But we will argue that such a response has a more complex character, representing a problematic amalgam of reactions to a set of taxing demands at a personal, disciplinary, and institutional level.

If one accepts that psychological and psychotherapeutic understandings are immersed in a historical process, then it has to be that new kinds of knowledge continually emerge as a result of theoretical, social, or even technological change. As new contexts arise, mental health institutions have a responsibility to foster exploration into diverse new areas. Disciplinary or psychotherapeutic modality groups, which may be said to "own" knowledge, must accommodate and explore these new contexts and the questions they throw up, authorize new knowledge extensions, or become moribund. Yet this need for a discipline to reach beyond itself can be fundamentally at odds with the institutionalized nature of disciplines and the organizations that represent the different therapeutic modalities. As such professional groups and networks form and elaborate; they of necessity build around themselves administrative and institutional superstructures that can become rigid and increasingly unable to adapt to new contexts. From the perspective of an anthropologist struggling to work in conjunction with economists, Harriss notes that

"Discipline" . . . produces the conditions for cumulation of knowledge and deepening of understanding of the physical and social worlds. But it is also clear that "discipline" is constraining and that it may be pushed to the point where it limits thought (and so becomes constraining and even repressive rather than productive). [Harriss, 2002, p. 1]

For Harriss, working *against* the disciplinary grain is essential for intellectual health:

Disciplines, like other kinds of sects, may be characterised by "religiosity", when particular practices or ways of acting come to be venerated in themselves, and others treated as quite unacceptable for no other reason than that they do not conform to the currently accepted canon. . . . The development of knowledge and understanding requires both "discipline" in the key sense of "instruction and exercise" that inculcates the system of rules, and a healthy disrespect for particular systems of rules when they stand in the way of the pursuit of knowledge. [Harriss, 2002, p. 1]

It is sometimes said, carelessly, that different psychotherapeutic modalities operate within different "paradigms". Perhaps we are used to thinking of the early-twentieth-century stand-offs between biological psychiatry, psychoanalysis, and behaviourism, believing that very different epistemologies are at work when mental disorder is under consideration: incommensurable norms of reasoning, causality, and truth. But do different therapeutic approaches differ so fundamentally? Is translation from the language of one into the language of the other so problematic? Does divergence in notions about how one comes to formulate a client's difficulties, how theory is developed, or how the idea of "evidence" is understood mean that we are condemned to misunderstand the reasoning within other modalities?

This seems unlikely; indeed, the fact that we can detect differences already presupposes a large degree of consensus, a common coordinate system on which to plot the different discursive positions. But it is only by making the effort to translate that we will come to a better realization of where and for whom sticking points are perceived to be. Consider Bolton and Hill's (2003) bravura account of parallels between a Freudian conception of intrapsychic defences and a post-empiricist conception of scientific theories.[2] There is real excitement in thinking about how a consideration of the points of difference between these conceptualizations may tell us something important about each and about their application in our work.

From many standpoints, lay and expert, mental health disciplines are seen to substantially claim the *same* subject matter and suffer only from being unwilling to share their knowledge easily and generously and to collaborate. Certainly, the two key models in the Tavistock and Portman share an orientation to the significance of relationships for how mental distress and disturbance emerge and develop, and to a recognition of

how disturbed individuals, communities or institutions may impact upon the minds and functioning of those engaged with them, or ... the manner in which teams and organisations can come to act in manners determined by their work and the relationships that constitute such work. [Lemma & Patrick, 2010, p. 6]

But despite such important shared positions, what tends to be emphasized in this Trust are the differences: differences not only in the
guiding theoretical concepts and key forms of practice, but also in the
relationship to theory, to tradition, and to the idea of change.

Family systems thinking sustains an insistent emphasis that a
person's life is not merely coloured, but radically shaped, by the values and beliefs associated with his or her wider community and the
prevailing power structures of gender, class, and race. Systemic therapists constantly work to theorize the social in explanatory accounts
of clients' intimate lives, to elaborate the way in which subjectivities
are formed within familial processes and relationships and the way
in which the social and cultural are played out in these processes and
relationships. This broadly post-positivist and social construction-
ist epistemology is also influential, however, for clinicians working
within other models. Some psychodynamic practitioners acknowledge that

> subjectivities are racialised, they are genderised, they are laced
> with the context of culture and epoch, and these phenomena con-
> stitute forms of identity and forms of difference that are power-
> fully multi-dimensional. [Harris, 2005, p. 1090]

Like systemic therapists, some psychodynamic practitioners may also
be committed to the view that social and psychological theories, far
from mirroring a reality independent of them, partly define and form
that reality and, importantly, can transform it by getting people to
articulate their actions and feelings in new ways (Fairfield, Layton, &
Stack, 2002). From this standpoint all theories are seen as contingent,
with people invested in them for complex reasons; as therapists, we
would accept the "complex unsettledness" (Harris, 2005) of our central theoretical constructs, to a point where, as Mitchell wryly notes,
"it sometimes appears that the capacity to contain the dread of not
knowing is a measure of clinical virtue; the fewer the convictions, the
braver and the better" (Mitchell, 1993, p. 43).

Of course this emphasis on different models as provisional, socially
situated templates for understanding some portion of human experience, the stress on the *ethics* of the therapeutic encounter in balance
with the *technical*, is for many cognitive, psychoanalytic, and indeed
family therapy clinicians profoundly wrong. For these more traditionally minded professionals, therapeutic equipoise is a hollow creed;
the need for certified, rigorous expert knowledge remains important,

with the different disciplines or modalities seen as offering completely contrasting skills, often in competition, for formulating clients' problems and providing solutions to them. Thus it is that splits can occur *among* modalities, as much as they can *between* them.

Whether one sees the different modalities as operating according to incommensurable and competing logics or as sharing a common thought-space, the fact is that the phenomena with which we grapple—mental distress and disturbance—exhibit a degree of complexity that our current models can hardly encompass. Multilayered and multidimensional explanations are required, and it seems foolish to take intellectual sides too vehemently. We need to develop our preferred models for their capacity to illuminate certain dimensions of experience, unpack certain processes, and analyse certain occurrences and observations. Yet we also need to somehow hold in mind alternative or additional theories in the human and natural sciences as relevant to our quest to understand and intervene in the forms of distress and disorder that present to us.

Multidisciplinarity, cross-disciplinarity, interdisciplinarity: what inhibits collaboration?

What forms of collaboration might we imagine? We are all familiar with *multidisciplinary* teams in mental health. These usually involve a non-integrative mixing in which each discipline or modality retains its methodologies and assumptions without mutual change or development. Typically, the key question in multidisciplinary teams is how well a clinical problem facing the group can be unpacked into separable subparts and then addressed via the distributed knowledge in the team. This is certainly the extent of collaborative work at many mental health institutions. Knowledge from more than one discipline is drawn on, but the disciplinary identity of each is preserved. While principles and practices are not held to be directly in contradiction, boundaries nevertheless remain firm. One discipline typically emerges as dominant in any interpretative enterprise. This kind of multidisciplinarity can be a benign and comfortable stance, or it can amount to no more than working in parallel and in bad grace. There is always the danger of rigidity and stereotyping, with defensiveness precluding a really thoughtful response to the other's ideas.

A more thoroughgoing *cross-disciplinary* form of collaboration aims to illuminate the subject of one discipline from the perspective of another. It rejects the old multidisciplinary paradigm of highly bound-aried traditions and half-hearted collaboration and makes a bolder attempt to negotiate meaning, with encouragement for the expression of differences and the articulation and open questioning of assump-tions. There is genuine curiosity about how one set of ideas could be theorized and perhaps made operative within another tradition. From this position we can imagine the emergence of fruitful innova-tions—new questions and new interventions—in full awareness of differences. One example in child-focused work is the new respect among child psychotherapists for empirical research in developmen-tal psychology and cognitive neuroscience (Music, 2010). Here the test of genuine cross-disciplinary respect will be whether empirical research is valued not just because it bolsters certain cherished psy-choanalytic conceptualizations of infant and childhood experience, but also because it interrogates them—and, of course, whether the empirical science allows itself to be influenced and challenged by clinical forms of knowing.

This kind of cross-disciplinarity may be especially relevant where the subject matter is felt to have been neglected, or where it cannot be adequately understood from a single disciplinary perspective—such as the impact of trauma, severe developmental disorders, or serious forms of eating or behavioural pathology. Such cross-disciplinary alliances can bring different kinds of science and clinical practice into conjunction, as well as direct attention to neglected of issues of power and culture.

Beyond cross-disciplinarity of this kind, deep *interdisciplinary* relationships (Hulme & Toye, 2005) that blend the practices and assumptions of two or more disciplines seem more elusive still. Here clinicians try to connect and more fully integrate several modalities in the pursuit of a common task. Interdisciplinary collaborators adopt a perspective unique to the collaborative effort and distinct from those of the cooperating disciplines, creating a new hybrid field. In such work—if the interdisciplinary effort can be sustained—the bounda-ries are re-drawn, and an overarching and coherent conceptual frame-work may be forged. This is a radical stance, threatening existing allegiances and identities but perhaps offering opportunities for a re-alignment of interest groups. In turn, deep interdisciplinary initiatives support the development of each contributing group by helping to make the implicit foundations of its discourse explicit. There are some in our field who believe that only such newly forged, integrated academic and professional disciplines will provide adequate answers in the future to the taxing intellectual questions that perplex and confound us.

The anxiety of influence and other fears

Let us return to the question of what makes a collaborative mindset so elusive. Fear of cross-disciplinarity may, we believe, reflect the "anxiety of influence".[3] By this we mean the unwillingness to acknowledge the way other traditions have played a part in the development of our preferred models. Attempts to remind ourselves of the "mongrel" nature of much of psychotherapy's theoretical heritage and the theoretically nomadic career of some of its leading figures can arouse worry that the intellectual integrity of our theoretical position is under attack. There is a fear of mopping up too many diverse influences and creating an unpalatable theoretical "soup". In preference, ideas and theories are often reconstructed retrospectively as having a clear and unambiguous story of development. The current threat of new and unfamiliar, but influential, modalities gaining favour with our public-health paymasters can further steel us to commit to disciplinary narratives of exclusion and self-sufficiency.

This purist position also confers on the holders the mantle of specialness, in full flight from the "ordinary", the bog-standard. We may believe that, if others have difficulty understanding our specialist language or the point of our therapeutic techniques, this only serves to establish the credentials of our model. It is often the case in the professional world that the wider the gap between the highly specialist ways of speaking and thinking associated with our disciplinary knowledge, the greater the perceived status of the professional.[4]

A modality's angry defence of the self-sufficient integrity of its core ideas can mask another anxiety: that its members lack the capacity for innovation and in particular—in the current context—for developing bold, short-term profitable new treatments for the therapeutic marketplace. A passionate attachment to historically sanctioned ideas may make it difficult for an individual or an institution to host the development of popular new interventions and may serve as a proud excuse for the failure to do so. New treatments typically bring elements from different models together in new ways, creating a different therapeutic style and idiom with only a faint nod towards its theoretical forebears. Significant innovation originates from outside, or between, disciplines at least as often as it originates from within them. To try to develop a new integrative model in a setting where pride in therapeutic "purity" is strong threatens to unsettle hegemonic claims.

Other anxieties emerge when collaborative therapy ventures seem to assume implicitly that the operation of "common factors" (e.g. Messer & Wampold, 2002) explains the success of our work, that the *shared* characteristics of our clinical practice are the effective elements. If a systems approach can be trusted to be as useful for a couple in conflict as a psychodynamic or cognitive approach, it might be because the specialist techniques are nothing other than a vehicle for mobilizing powerful, common change processes. If we entertain this possibility, we are implying that each modality's distinct knowledge base, evolved over time, may need be re-evaluated. Similarities have also been highlighted through the process of manualization of therapeutic activity, itself a consequence of the shift to evidence-based practice. By stripping the professional language of descriptions of therapeutic activity and translating ideas into a more everyday shared vocabulary, similarities across approaches become more identifiable. We might begin to wonder whether the specialist techniques are only a means for keeping the therapist engaged and enthusiastic, harnessing the power of therapist conviction and hope. Perhaps a common sensibility is at work in all effective therapists. And perhaps there are processes in effective therapy that no modality theorizes adequately.

It is worth considering whether being a provider of core psychotherapy training has a particular role in locking clinicians into a more unanimous, un-conflicted, even heroic account of their tradition, under an obligation to pass on a corpus of certain and secure knowledge in an unambiguous and forthright way. Qualifying-level trainees often expect a grounding in the work of a pantheon of revered figures from the past, as if this were a marker of a mature discipline. Canguilhem (1968) describes the ways in which scientific disciplines tend to identify themselves partly through a certain conception of their history: what he calls "a sanctioned" past. Rose shows the way this history is typically arranged

> in a more or less continual sequence, as that which led to the present and anticipated it, that virtuous tradition of which the present is the inheritor. It is a past of genius, of precursors, of influences, of obstacles overcome, crucial experiments, discoveries and the like. [Rose, 1996, p. 3]

The danger for a training institution can be that it increasingly attracts trainees who desire this version of a clinical tradition, associated with a mono-disciplinary model of mental disorder and its remedies, and discourages trainees who might want to move more freely between different disciplinary cultures. Such a culture will be at odds with the recent development of competency frameworks (Roth & Pilling, 2007) for practitioners who are not trained in a single therapeutic model.

Alongside this defence of revered traditions may sit an anxiety that our personal attachment to our core models—the personal relevance and meaning of these models in our own lives—is no longer a defensible element in our preference for one mode of working over another. For many therapists it is a steadfast belief in a relatively unchanging model that bestows the confidence to hold fast in the face of confusing and unbearable distress. Campbell, who developed the work of systemic family therapy at the Tavistock for 30 years, wrote that

> The nature of the work, calling on our own emotional reservoirs, or having unwanted feelings and behaviours projected into us, requires an unshakeable conviction that we posses an equally powerful force—our own belief system, which will enable us to survive. [Campbell, 1998]

The modern NHS, in its reverence for evidence-based treatments, can seem to ignore the crucial role played by passion and emotion in securing clinician allegiance to one model over another (Cooper, 2008). And, of course, there is also likely to be an unconscious element in our attachments to our preferred modality. Stokes (1994) suggests that psychiatrists operate with a need to deny dependency, responding to their own experience of prolonged institutionalized dependency in their own training; other therapists, he argues, idealize the therapist–client relationship, "remaining endlessly 'glued' together as if the generation of hope about the future were by itself a cure" (p. 26). Any call to surrender some of the certainties of one's therapeutic allegiance may be felt as a significant loss.

The art of mis-meeting

We believe that together these represent some of the anxieties that may lead psychotherapists to develop a backward-looking narrative characterized by metaphors of pure/impure and strong/diluted applied to ideas and the notion of insider/outsider applied to fellow clinicians. Such exclusive disciplinary or institutional narratives tend to evolve in relation to stories told about rivals or adversaries. Disciplinary religiosity requires a clearly defined, clearly maligned other. Baumann writes about how the creation of a "we" involves a delimitation of a "them"—the determination of an "other" to play the role of the outsider:

> Only by crystallizing and solidifying what they are not (and what they do not wish to be, or what they would not say they are) into the counter-image of the enemies, may the friends assert what they are, what they want to be and what they want to be thought of as being. [Baumann, 1991, p. 53]

To turn advocates of another modality into the "other" often involves resorting to ill-informed mutual criticism based on anecdotes of misunderstood or atypical episodes. Where an alliance *is* struck between advocates of different models of psychotherapeutic intervention, the friendship is often formed in opposition to a hostile other.

For psychological therapists in many mental health settings, the "other" has traditionally been conventional psychiatric practice (Lemma & Patrick, 2010), characterized as obsession with diagnosis, pharmacological interventions, and non-intentional explanations. For psychotherapists, such a clear and time-honoured enemy is comfortably recognized in an adversarial contest that can serve to bolster the identity of each adversary. But this conventional enemy in mental health has to some extent lost intellectual power. In sophisticated circles, traditional psychiatry is increasingly discredited (Bentall, 2009) or seen as being limited in the application of its knowledge and expertise (Bolton, 2008). For many psychotherapists, the newer enemy is the advocate of a cognitive approach, whose recent success has taken many by surprise and who has turned out to be a determined opponent. But if dialogue was limited in the settled adversarial world of known enemies, it has become even more limited in this new competitive world where, in the United Kingdom, the National Institute for Health and Clinical Excellence (NICE) rules. In the mental health wars, cognitive therapies are, in Baumann's terms, the "strangers", the newcomers who arouse confusion and perturbation and who must be treated with disdain. Many psychotherapists struggle to take cognitive therapy seriously as a therapeutic approach, and myths abound about what cognitive therapists think and do: their work is held to be completely formulaic and rule-bound; they are said to take no account of the individuality of the client; therapist subjectivity is treated as a nuisance factor, and so on. Caricaturing of this kind perfects "the art of mis-meeting":

> Intercourse with the stranger is always an incongruity. . . . It is best not to meet strangers at all. As one cannot really keep away from the space they occupy or share, the next best solution is a meeting that is not really a meeting, a meeting pretending not to be one. . . . The art of mis-meeting is first and foremost a set of techniques that serve to de-ethicalise the relationship with the stranger . . . denying the stranger moral significance. [Baumann, 1993, p. 153]

This art of mis-meeting—this denial of the humanity and comprehensibility of the "stranger"—works against the possibility for dialogue and, ultimately, for adaptation and innovation.

We believe that open processes of contest and rivalry between different traditions, embodying different values, are part of the constitutive nature of antagonism in social life, a condition about which the political theorist Mouffe has written vividly. For Mouffe, the moral and political significance of contest and struggle, conflict and passion cannot be overstated. Tensions can be negotiated, precarious solutions can be articulated, but elimination of the antagonism can never be a reasonable aim. Acceptance of "a plurality of just answers" (Mouffe, 2000a) is the necessary condition for a democratic society. According to this view, agonistic confrontation, far from jeopardizing valuable processes of decision-making, is the very condition of its existence. A well-functioning institution will therefore be characterized by vibrant clashes of passionately held positions. Only at times of extreme crisis is there a danger that the presence of the Other might be perceived as a negation of one's own identity (Mouffe, 1993).

Writing from a cultural theory perspective, Thompson (2006) also sees this kind of conflict in any policy process as "endemic, inevitable and desirable, rather than pathological, curable or deviant". He cites the influence of Schapiro (1988), who coined the term "clumsy institutions" as a way of escaping from the idea that, when we are faced with contradictory definitions of a problem and solution, we must choose one and reject the rest.

> Clumsiness emerges as preferable to elegance (optimising around just one of the definitions of the problem and, in the process, silencing the other voices) once we realise that what looks like irreconcilable contradiction is, in fact, essential contestation. [Thomson, 2006, p. 232]

Allowing different models to have a strong and legitimate voice in an institution means committing to the belief that the liveliness of its culture rests on the possibilities for dialogue, and that from such dialogue creative developments will emerge.

Organizational change:
the rules of the democratic game

Of the many modalities in the current NHS mental health economy, none can have the last word on the future of mental health treatment. In our mental health institutions we should welcome the frank argumentation that arises when clinicians shape a set of collective identities around clearly differentiated positions and are supported to articulate their argumentative positions. We need to hear from those who emphasize therapist knowledge and authority about the mind and its structures, from those who explore unconscious elements of emotional life, from those who pay special attention to the constraining effect of the actually existing conditions of clients' lives, from serious practitioners of brief evidence-based models, and from experts on the science of outcomes and effectiveness. And, in addition, we need people voicing the suspicion that it is power rather than reasoning that is at stake in debates between these diverse modalities. If one of these viewpoints is ignored or dismissed, it will eventually force its way back onto the agenda. At some point, one disciplinary discourse will appear to "win" the conversation and so get to dictate the terms of debate for a while. Then the power shifts again, new voices are heard or old ones listened to afresh, experiences are re-described, and explanations reconfigured, in new or revitalized vocabularies.

What is required at the organizational level for a range of different modalities and cross-disciplinary attempts to be heard, taken seriously, and brought "compulsively" into connection?

1. The institutional leadership needs to believe that no theoretical approach is all-encompassing, no knowledge is exhaustive. At the top there needs to be an acknowledgement that there is a dimension of undecidability between the leading therapy models, a disavowal of the notion of "universal" systems of thought whose aim is to arrive at a single, stable account of mental life and relational processes. An institution that supports genuinely collaborative cross-disciplinary work must believe that no modality represents anything more than a partial, tentative, and fallible account of the world it purports to explain. This surrender of claims to certainty and necessity can be painful:

> Crusading truths los[e] their power to humiliate but they also forfeit much of their past ability to offer the succour . . . that truths used to lavish on the converted. [Baumann, 1991, p. 251]

We can claim that the knowledge in our tradition is satisfying, useful, elegant, productive, even that it fits the fact as we see them. But there is no point external to all models from which we can offer a universal judgement, a stamp of authoritative confirmation. There can be no "solace of closure" (Hall, 1991).

2. An organization needs many occasions where disagreement—and hostility—can be shaped and its destructive potential diffused. For a start, there have to be adequate settings where different disciplines or modalities are present and available for dialogue and debate. This work needs to happen in small enough groups with sufficient regularity for real articulation of positions—not parodies—to take place. We need to be wary of simplifications and acknowledge that each member of staff has multiple affiliations or identities, which are important for his or her self-definition. And there must be agreement as to the rules of the democratic game. Mouffe (2000b) reminds us that rules are not neutral procedures: they assume substantial ethical commitments. Rules in plural or "clumsy" institutions must signify a determination to confront professional conceit and unhelpful group dynamics and to dismantle the structures that allow them to flourish.

3. Institutions must resolutely challenge any assumption that the world views of the different modalities are incommensurable. People must be encouraged to work to make their meanings plain, to unpack

the givens of their approach in language that can be readily understood by "outsiders", and to use specialized language only where a
term or concept is genuinely unavailable in ordinary parlance. As
specialists, we should all be under pressure to share the wisdom of
our approaches, to lend our knowledge, to scaffold others' grasp of
our best ideas through sustained dialogue. This means paying attention to the actual detail of our cross-modal transactions to reveal and
understand the intricate and uncertain process of negotiation. Some
staff may be better at taking on the hermeneutic work of "translating"
across languages, turning the unfamiliar into the familiar and excising
jargon, and they should be valued for this talent.

4. Each discipline or modality may make its own accommodation to meet the external demands for manualization, brief-treat-
ment models, and the quantification of outcomes. But this process
of accommodation should not back us into our disciplinary corners.
Rather, we should be drawn to share what we feel is non-negotiable
in our approaches. We should make opportunities to spell out which
technical or theoretical commitments in our modalities must survive
all pressure to reduce, to trim, to package, and to measure.

5. Taking these considerations seriously, accredited disciplinary
training courses should be obliged to introduce students to a sympathetic explication of at least one other model, to inculcate a critical
understanding of the science of "common factors" alongside the science of "evidence-supported treatments", and to promote an authentic
and energetic discussion of cross-disciplinarity in its many forms.

6. We need to make serious—and creatively playful—attempts
to combine or integrate modalities. This may be in the context of
working together in a service or on a case, or it might mean con-
ceiving multilayered, pioneering clinical interventions or professional trainings. The complex difficulties that arise across the age
range—such as couples engaged in intimate violence and their children, families where chronic disability or illness affect individuals
across time, the impact of abuse and trauma—are examples of work
where debate could be creative. Debate will focus on such questions
as: where are the points of tension and the points of outright disagreement, and how can they best be talked about? What is at stake
for the different professionals in deciding how to proceed? What is
being emphasized or privileged in each of the modalities, and what
is felt to be missing? Psychotherapy process research can help us

here with its curiosity about change processes in the talking therapies and how these may be better understood through close inspection of everyday client–therapist interchanges (e.g. Castonguay &
Beutler, 2006). It may be, as social researcher Pawson complains,
that "social science is a science like no other, deliver[ing] a curious knowledge base beset with inconsistency and rivalry" (Pawson,
2006, p. 1), but we might find ourselves united across the modality
divide in our surprise and occasional delight at the elegant findings
of high-quality, clinically meaningful research.

We do not underestimate the dangers. The emphasis on newly
minted brief interventions, the paring back of concepts and ideas,
the oversimplification of accepted knowledges for training purposes,
can underestimate the "indescribable"—the art of therapy and human
dialogue that is kept vibrant through intradiscipline conversations
and scholarship and that needs to be valued and preserved. The very
structure of disciplines that still exists within the NHS can provide a
check to threats to quality in service delivery and workforce development. We are far from advocating the abolition of disciplinary
difference, but we are trying to develop its generative rather than its
ossifying potential.

Mental health institutions like the Tavistock and Portman have a
public service commitment to strive for a better understanding of how
the different psychotherapeutic modalities are connected, to explore
what shared principles or processes link us in our diverse practices,
to look at how we most creatively combine ways of working, and
to engage in the critical debates that emerge when we consider our
differences. We can usefully and resourcefully argue for why one
approach is superior to another, not that it is superior for all time. The
challenge is to feel enough confidence in one's preferred model that
these ideas serve as a basis for action, while not needing these ideas
to be dominant, and to recognize the way that alternative models
do the same work for others. We have to manage the pull towards
arguments and dissension, splits and divisions, without breaking off
into destructive rivalry. This means that claims to epistemological
privilege need to be disabled and disciplinary priority brought to an
end. In all contexts where mental distress is evidenced and mental
well-being sought, we need new alliances where people step away
from complacency and dogma and start to evolve new connections,
new solutions, more "just answers".

Notes

1. Systemic psychotherapy was only officially accepted as a separate discipline, and the second key modality in the Trust, in 2002.

2. Bolton and Hill write: "Threats [e.g. to expectations of safety] can be denied representation, or they can be attacked and destroyed in thought. Satisfaction of needs can likewise be thought, even if not really achieved. Such strategies operate within the mind as opposed to reality: they are acts of the imagination, and they involve departure from or distortion of reality" (Bolton & Hill, 2003, p. 293). They then draw a parallel between this insight of Freud's and "the post-empiricist recognition that some intentional states constitute the core of belief, to be protected from counter-evidence, and the inevitable conclusion then that while such protection averts perceived catastrophe, it involves at least distortion of reality, and perhaps manifest disorder" (p. 292).

3. A free adaptation of the classicist and philosopher Allan Bloom's notion of what the "strong poet" fears (Bloom, 1973).

4. On these issues, see Till (2009) for the profession of architecture.

References

Baumann, Z. (1991). *Modernity and Ambivalence*. Cambridge: Polity Press.

Baumann, Z. (1993). *Postmodern Ethics*. Oxford: Blackwell.

Bentall, R. P. (2009). *Doctoring the Mind: Why Psychiatric Treatments Fail*. London: Allen Lane.

Bloom, A. (1973). *The Anxiety of Influence: A Theory of Poetry*. Oxford: Oxford University Press.

Bolton, D. (2008). *What Is Mental Disorder? An Essay In Philosophy, Science and Values*. Oxford: Oxford University Press.

Bolton, D., & Hill, J. (2003). *Mind, Meaning and Mental Disorder: The Nature of Causal Explanation in psychology and Psychiatry* (2nd edition). Oxford: Oxford University Press.

Campbell, D. (1998) (with Bell, D., Klauber, T., & Clulow, C.). *Ideas Which Divide the Tavistock: What Are They Really About?* [soundrecording]. Tavistock Centre Scientific Meeting, Tavistock Clinic, London (12 January).

Canguilhem, G. (1968). *Etudes d'histoire et de philosophie des sciences*. Paris: Vrin.

Castonguay, L. G., & Beutler, L. E. (2006). Principles of therapeutic change: A task force on participants, relationships, and techniques factors. *Journal of Clinical Psychology, 62* (6): 631–638.

Cooper, A. (2008). Interprofessional working: Choice or destiny? *Clinical Child Psychology and Psychiatry, 14* (4): 531–536.

Dicks, H. V. (1970). *Fifty Years of the Tavistock Clinic*. London: Routledge & Kegan Paul.

Fairfield, S., Layton, L., & Stack, C. (2002). *Bringing the Plague: Towards a Postmodern Psychoanalysis*. New York: Other Press.

Hall, S. (1991). On postmodernism and articulation: An interview with Stuart Hall. In: D. Morley & C. Kuan-Hsing (Eds.), *Stuart Hall: Critical Dialogues in Cultural Studies*. New York: Routledge.

Harris, A. (2005). Gender in linear and nonlinear history. *Journal of the American Psychoanalytic Association, 53*: 1079–1095.

Harriss, J. (2002). *The Case for Cross-Disciplinary Approaches in International Development*. Working Paper Series No. 02–23. London: London School of Economics.

Hulme, D., & Toye, J. (2005). *The Case for Cross-Disciplinary Social Science Research on Poverty, Inequality and Well-Being*. ESRC Global Poverty Research Group paper. Available at: http://economics.ouls.ox.ac .uk/14081/1/gprg-wps-001.pdf

Lemma, A., & Patrick, M. (2010). *Off the Couch: Contemporary Psychoanalytic Application*. Hove: Routledge.

Messer, S. B., & Wampold, B. E. (2002). Let's face facts: Common factors are more potent then specific therapy ingredients. *Clinical Psychology: Science and Practice, 9* (1): 21–25.

Mitchell, S. (1993). *Hope and Dread in Psychoanalysis*. New York: Basic Books.

Mouffe, C. (1993). Pluralism and modern democracy. In: *The Return of the Political*. London: Verso.

Mouffe, C. (2000a). Wittgenstein, political theory and democracy. In: *The Democratic Paradox*. London: Verso.

Mouffe, C. (2000b). *Deliberative Democracy or Agonistic Pluralism*. Political Science Series papers. Vienna: Institute for Advanced Studies.

Music, G. (2010). *Nurturing Natures: Attachment and Children's Emotional, Sociocultural and Brain Development*. Hove: Psychology Press.

Patrick, M. (2010). Psychoanalytic psychotherapy now. *Psychoanalytic Psychotherapy, 24* (1): 8–13.

Pawson, R. (2006). *Evidence-Based Policy: A Realist Perspective*. London: Sage.

Rose, N. (1996). Power and subjectivity: Critical history and psychology. In C. F. Grautmann & K. J. Gergen (Eds.), *Historical Dimensions of Psychological Discourse*. Cambridge: Cambridge University Press.

Roth, A., & Pilling, S. (2007). *The Competencies Required to Deliver Effective Cognitive Behavioural Therapy for People with Depression and with Anxiety Disorders*. Available at: www.ucl.ac.uk/CORE.

Schapiro, M. (1988). Judicial selection and the design of clumsy institutions. *Southern California Law Review, 61*: 1555–1569.

Stokes, J. (1994). The unconscious at work in groups and teams: Contributions from the work of Wilfred Bion. In: A. Obholzer & V. Z. Roberts (Eds.), *The Unconscious at Work*. London: Routledge.

Thompson, M. (2006). Cultural theory, cultural change and clumsiness. In: M. Verweij & M. Thompson (Eds.), *Clumsy Solutions for a Complex World*. Basingstoke: Palgrave Macmillan.

Till, J. (2009). *Architecture Depends*. Cambridge, MA: MIT Press.

PART II

PSYCHOANALYTIC INTERVENTIONS WITH YOUNG ADULTS AND ADULTS

Introduction

Alessandra Lemma

The world in which we live and work shapes how psychic distress is expressed. New social realities present us with challenges that impact on the mind: the decimation in many cultures of the extended family (geographical distances between relatives are now greater than at any other time in history), the widespread incidence of divorce, the reality of different familial configurations (such as reconstituted, homosexual, or single-parent families), fractured local communities, the impact of new reproductive technologies, of economic recession, and of climate change, to name but a few. In these new social and cultural contexts we are faced with an increase in certain clinical presentations, which, in turn, place different demands on mental health and social care staff working with some of our most challenging patients (see chapter six, by Carine Minne). The patients who are referred to mental health services nowadays are in these respects very different from those who crossed the threshold of the Tavistock Clinic in the 1920s.

Such phenomena also alert us to the "mental state" of our society. As mental health providers, it is not sufficient for us to respond in the clinical situation—our ideas and understanding of the mind should also be applied to intervening at the social level. In fact, I would go as far as to say that it is our moral duty to do so.

The ethnic diversity of our patients provides another dimension to the current landscape that mental health services need to address in order to ensure the accessibility and acceptability of their services. Providing help that is felt to be acceptable to patients from a variety of backgrounds requires us to revisit our service models and be prepared to make adaptations, as is well illustrated through the development of the Black People's Consultation Service (chapter four, by Linda Young & Frank Lowe).

Changing external landscapes also require us to revisit our theories. For example, irrespective of social background, nowadays most pre-pubescent children who live in urban areas dress and act more like adolescents. A kind of pseudo-sexuality is encouraged through social media and consumer culture, such that the very experience of the body and hence of sexuality has been redefined. From a psychoanalytic point of view this also raises the question of whether there is still a latency period in development (Guignard, 2008).

The changing face of clinical practice is striking when we consider not only the highly deprived backgrounds of some of the young people who present for help, but also the way their expectations and the consequent pressures on them have changed. One of the distinctive features of the work in this Trust, well captured by two of the chapters in this section (chapter three, by Stephen Briggs & Louise Lyon, and chapter four, by Linda Young & Frank Lowe), is the way that the needs of adolescents and young adults have been responded to in a developmentally appropriate manner through a dedicated service for this age group. Adolescence as a stage of life, and the adolescent process that drives it—a qualitatively distinctive state of mind—calls for interventions that manage to respect the young person's striving towards independence and the regressive pull of childhood longings that mobilizes infantile anxieties.

If we are thinking about the world in which young people are growing up today, the impact of virtual reality on psychic and social functioning deserves particular mention. "Playing" in cyberspace may serve to bypass the arduous psychic task required to represent experience, giving way instead to simulation, with the attendant risk that the fake can replace the real and become more compelling. At the same time these very same technological developments, which can be "mis"-used, invite us to consider novel ways of reaching greater numbers of people in psychological distress—for example, through online therapeutic interventions that are informed by a psychoanalytic understanding of individual and group processes (see chapter nine, by Richard Graham). These external forces, which have in some instances also brought about invaluable developments, such as the possibilities afforded by virtual reality, need to be integrated into how we understand clinical presentations. What we see and hear in the clinical situation tells the story of an individual, couple, or family and their relationships, but it is also a current, running commentary on the society in which we live.

Another way of putting all this is that we are faced with increasing layers of complexity alongside the uncertainty of our social structures, both in our everyday lives and also at the clinical level. This complexity is especially apparent in work with young people who are confronted with seemingly endless possibilities for reinvention as self-identity has become far more deliberative (Featherstone, 2000; Giddens, 1991). Modernity has freed us from the idea that birth is destiny, and we are invited, for example, to see our bodies as negotiable works-in-progress (Lemma, 2010) with the attendant pressures this may place on vulnerable young people—and adults—who struggle to integrate their sexual body into their self-image (Laufer & Laufer, 1984).

"Complexity" as a feature of a clinical presentation is hard to define (see, for example, chapter five, by Brian Rock & Anca Carrington). Moreover, as is well illustrated by the clinical work described in this book, it cannot be thought of solely as the property of an individual patient: it is also, always, the property of a particular system. Indeed, a distinctive feature of how this institution approaches complexity is that it is viewed as an inevitable condition of being human and of human systems, of which our organizations are a prime example.

Patients who are seen to present a challenge to services appear to constitute a distinct group in terms of a greater number of more severe problems, a greater and more negative impact on services and on individual clinicians, and a more negative perception by staff, and they receive a poorer service (Davies, 2008; see also chapter six, by Carine Minne). Complexity, however, is often a way of naming the practitioner's "difficult" feelings about the patient that cannot be recognized, acknowledged, or understood. In responding to complexity, it becomes essential to focus on clinician- *and* service-based factors, not least keeping in mind that no therapeutic modality holds the key to "managing complexity". If we truly want to help those with mental health problems and respond to the complexity of the problems we are confronted with, then our services thus need to reflect therapeutic plurality and multidisciplinarity. The importance of the latter is inscribed in the fabric of this institution, with all departments bringing together doctors, nurses, psychologists, child and adult psychotherapists, and social workers, as will be apparent in the pages of this book, and of the subsequent two volumes that follow. In relation to the work with adults and young adults, this work is primarily (even if not exclusively) rooted in, or informed by, psychoanalytic ideas—that is, by a receptivity to an unconscious mind as it is manifest in the life of the individual, the couple (see chapter seven, by Joanna Rosenthall), and the group.

References

Davies, F. (2008). *New Ways (and Means) of Working and Delivering Care to Meet Complex Needs*. Paper presented at the 2008 Psychological Therapies in the NHS Conference, London, October.

Featherstone, M. (Ed.) (2000). *Body Modification*. London: Sage.

Giddens, A. (1991). *Modernity and Self Identify*. Cambridge: Polity Press.

Guignard, S. (2008). Envy in Western society: Today and tomorrow. In: P. Roth & A. Lemma (Eds.), *Envy and Gratitude Revisited*. London: Karnac.

Laufer, M., & Laufer, E. (1984). *Adolescence and Developmental Breakdown*. New Haven, CT: Yale University Press.

Lemma, A. (2010). Copies without originals: The psychodynamics of cosmetic surgery. *Psychoanalytic Quarterly, 79* (1): 129–157.

CHAPTER THREE

Time-limited psychodynamic psychotherapy for adolescents and young adults

Stephen Briggs & Louise Lyon

This chapter discusses processes involved in articulating and evaluating a model of time-limited psychodynamic psychotherapy for young people, developed in the Adolescent Department in a multidisciplinary team working in a specialist service for young people with mental health difficulties. Time-limited therapeutic approaches are increasingly deployed in contemporary mental health practice, which recognizes an increased role for psychological therapies. These therapeutic modalities are largely—if not entirely—time-limited and focus on short-term relief of symptoms and problem behaviours. In contrast, this model of time-limited psychodynamic psychotherapy has at its core a treatment that focuses on the emotional and relational aspects of the adolescent developmental process. It aims to be relevant for contemporary practice in mental health services, to be replicable and evidence-based and usable within current resource availabilities. It aims also to provide a critical perspective to therapeutic modalities for adolescents that are symptom-oriented and practices that are diagnostically and risk-management-led, particularly through connecting the psychological processes of therapy with the social contexts for contemporary adolescents through the developmentally focused approach. The model is in a state of evolution, and the discussion here will, first, identify some key contexts for the development of time-limited psychodynamic psychotherapy and, second, illustrate aspects of the model, including the role of audit, manualization, and the relationship between process and outcome. An illustrative case example is used to closely follow therapeutic processes in this approach for young people of different ages and hence at different points in the adolescent process.

Psychoanalytic time-limited therapy

This model of time-limited psychodynamic psychotherapy draws on and adapts a distinguished history of brief or time-limited psychoanalytic therapy, a history that is often in the shadow of the predominant open-ended method. Time-limited psychoanalytic therapy began, *ad hoc*, with Freud's occasional brief interventions and his imposition of a time limit on the treatment of the Wolf Man (Freud, 1918b [1914]), to the latter's dismay and disbelief. Modern applications are found in the work of Mann (1973), Malan and Osimo (1992), Davanloo (2000), Shefler (1993), Charman (2004), Coren (2009), and Lemma, Target, and Fonagy (chapter ten, this volume). Psychodynamic brief therapies have some core features: focus for treatment based on a psychodynamic formulation, emphasis on ending that begins with the decision to use a time limit, and applying psychoanalytic therapeutic techniques, including emphasis on depth and use of the transference. There is debate about whether techniques need to change, to be more intensive (Davanloo, 2000) or not, and about the selection of cases that are suitable for briefer interventions. Malan (1976), for example, argued that problems at the Oedipal rather than pre-Oedipal level are more suitable. Schefler considers that "the most critical patient attribute is the strength of the ego and its capacity to allow rapid affective involvement and equally rapid affective disengagement" (2000, p. 90). Clearly for brief therapies the aims of psychotherapy need to be aligned with the timescale and be more modest than those for longer term therapies (Holmes, 1998). There needs to be a distinction between brief methods designed to meet particular therapeutic aims and objectives, for specific populations of service users, and those that are pragmatically organized around resource restrictions within services.

Brief therapy and adolescence

The qualities of change and transition that are central to adolescence suggest that young people may constitute a group for whom brief or time-limited psychodynamic psychotherapy is suitable, and it is perhaps surprising that there are not more examples available of such models being developed. However, it is also true there are few models of time-limited therapy for adolescents in any therapeutic modality, and this may reflect widely perceived difficulties in engaging and sustaining adolescents in therapy (Baruch, 2001).

It has been suggested that one aspect of this difficulty is the gap between young people and adults with regard to the perception of time (Shefler, 2000). For some adolescents, even a short-term intervention can seem entrapping and endless. For others, the notion of a time limit can seem like an oppressive imposition on freedom. Therefore, assessment of suitability for time-limited psychotherapy depends primarily on an understanding of the meaning of the developmental process for each individual adolescent, in relation to both internal processes and social contexts.

Radically changed social contexts for young people generate new and different psychological tasks and require specific qualities to negotiate transitions that are extended, less structured, and more uncertain (Briggs, 2009). There are increased pressures to think flexibly about future plans and pathways and to develop narratives that make sense of these experiences (Walkerdine, Lucey, & Melody, 2001). Distinct transitional points in educational terms—exams, at 16 and 18 and at university—for increasing numbers of young people—provide a focus for testing readiness to meet developmental challenges.

Pathways into adulthood have become more complex. While psychoanalytic thinking has richly theorized the development from puberty into adolescence, there has been less written about the way that adolescents move into adulthood. The realities of the imminence of the need to engage with external realities have often propelled late adolescents into therapy, when they have to face the immediacy of decisions, to take up careers, form partnerships, leave home (Waddell, 1998). In current social contexts, the external factors often create a deeply contradictory situation: young people may be psychologically ready to leave home, take up a career, enter a partnership, but they continue to depend on parental support. It is more realistic to see adolescents moving into adulthood in a piecemeal or uneven ways, becoming positioned as "more adult" in particular domains, relationships, employment, becoming a parent (Briggs, 2008). Developing subjectivity in particular domains of experience more accurately describes these changes than does the more traditional concept of identity formation. There are "fast-" and "slow-"track routes into adulthood (Jones, 2006), with different consequences and associated difficulties. The slow-track route involves a delayed transition to adulthood, longer time spent—often through the twenties—in semi-independent relatedness to parents—including financial dependency—and deferred work or career roles. The uncertainties of the slow-track route can arouse anxieties and be difficult to bear. On the other hand, fast-track routes can lead to premature taking up of adult roles—often by the most disadvantaged young people—with risks of social exclusion, marginalization, and lack of education, training, and work.

Psychoanalytic therapy provides opportunities for linking the internal, individual, relational, and social aspects of the process of adolescence, recognizing key transitional markers and the ways these are experienced individually. Time-limited psychodynamic therapy also presents opportunities for providing structure and focus within the therapy where these are socially absent, confusing, or concentrated on one particular aspect of experience.

Time-limited psychotherapy: the model

This model of time-limited therapy is rooted in, and adapts an established model of, psychodynamic psychotherapy for young people. This model has been articulated over some years in the Tavistock's Adolescent Department. We will briefly describe some of the key contributions. Bird (1987, 1989) identified that assessing adolescents involves the question of identifying to whom pain and anxiety belong and are attributed. This recognizes the importance of projective processes in adolescence and that pain, concern, or worry about an adolescent in difficulty may be located within the adolescent or within someone else, usually a parent or carer, in the adolescent's network. Williams (1978) explored the dynamic meaning of depression in adolescence—as a force for development as well as a painful situation—and the emotional impact on the therapist of working with the adolescent process. Anderson and Dartington (1998) defined the adolescent process as follows:

> If the adolescent is to successfully achieve adulthood, he [sic] must re-negotiate every aspect of his relationship with himself, and with his external and internal objects in a new context—this activity is what we often refer to as the adolescent process. It is like a review of the life that has been lived so far . . . all adolescents have to deal with the experience of being out of balance to some extent. Indeed it seems to be those young people who have the inner strength and resources to bear to continue the experience of being naturally out of balance, as well as an environment which can support this, who can achieve the best adjustment in adult life [Anderson & Dartington, 1998, p. 3]

Waddell (1999, 2002) has elaborated the process of assessing the qualities of anxiety and psychic pain within the context of adolescent development, the "extraordinary entanglement, in the adolescent's world, of internal and external, and of bodily and mental forces and factors" (2002, p. 367). She also discussed the role of narcissism in adolescent development as an "adolescent organization" (Waddell, 2006), part of the developmental process rather than a diagnostic category indicating pathology as in adults, and this points to the necessity to refrain from premature judgement about adolescent difficulties. She comments on "the swiftness with which what seem to be deeply entrenched narcissistic structures may be modified or modulated in response to even quite small internal or external change" (Waddell, 2006, p. 23).

Binding together all these approaches over time is the underpinning view that adolescence provides, in the words of Blos (1962), a "second chance", that there is potential for growth and the reorganization of the internal world. This notion has gathered support from recent neuroscientific studies showing that changes to the brain at puberty have an effect on cognition, affect regulation, learning, and memory; in adolescence, the brain shows "greater neural plasticity" (Patton & Viner, 2007, p. 1132). The flexibility supports—but also, at times, inhibits—developmental processes of re-evaluation.

Based on this model of the adolescent process, therapeutic practices with adolescents involve distinctive techniques and require different approaches from working with children or with adults. In particular, the process of engagement of the adolescent means taking account of a tension between being dependent and more separate, the projection of intense feelings and the possibility of providing a space to see if and how the adolescent attends therapy. Can she or he get her/himself there and take up the offer of an individual space, or not—or, if there is less separateness between parent and adolescent, do parent and adolescent come together and wish to be seen together?

To fit this approach, a method of assessment consisting of four sessions over four consecutive weeks has been established as a means of engaging the adolescent in therapy, through providing an experience of what being in therapy might feel like—coming once a week, experiencing this kind of relatedness—and also of demonstrating the processes of thinking and negotiability that are central to the process:

> Conducting an assessment over a period of a few weeks offers some opportunity to test the strength of the impetus that first brings a young person to the clinic; to discover whether that impetus really came from him or herself; to see whether it is possible to hold on to trains of thought and emotional links over periods of separation and to foster a relationship with a therapist, which could be a thinking one and not a "dumping" one. [Waddell, 1999, p. 224]

Therapists will have in mind adolescents' anxieties about being in therapy, and they will be prepared to spend time recognizing and talking about this, as well as aiming to identify the qualities of the specific anxiety brought by each individual adolescent. Maintaining the adolescent in therapy thus focuses on containing anxiety about the process through, on the one hand, talking about the structure of the therapy and the thinking of the therapist and, on the other hand, aiming to understand deep anxieties stirred up by the process of starting therapy and the difficulties that have brought the young person to therapy. The therapeutic process itself focuses on the relationship between therapist and adolescent and links this with formulations of difficulties in the adolescent process; the therapist aims to find ways, through interpretation and containment, of making sense of these with the adolescent patient.

This model of an assessment phase of four meetings has been applied to time-limited therapy and very brief therapy (Lyon, 2004). Assessment of suitability for time-limited therapy and identification of a developmentally based focus are part of this process. The treatment phase consists of 16 weekly sessions, ideally by the same clinician who undertakes the assessment. A total of 16 sessions was decided as the length partly because this mapped on to other models of time-limited therapy and also through reflecting on what was experienced as a helpful time length. A review meeting can take place around 4–6 weeks after the treatment.

Suitability for time-limited therapy is a crucial and complex issue, requiring a psychosocial assessment to understand both internal and external factors and the interaction between these. Anxieties about the key social transition points can often trigger a young person to seek therapeutic help—or to organize others into seeking this on her/his behalf. However, the external factor is not usually enough on its own to justify an offer of time-limited therapy; it is important to link external time frames with internal factors. These can include adolescents' fears of entrapment in an open-ended therapy, the need for a structured approach to therapeutic involvement, and recognizing the anxieties young people may have about being involved with and becoming dependent on another adult while the developmental process is impelling them towards greater independence. It is important to assess how the young person responds to the experience of separating from the therapy at the end of each session; thus, assessment is concerned not only with the capacity to engage, but also with the potential to be able to leave.

The 16 sessions of time-limited psychodynamic psychotherapy are based on three key principles: (1) working with a developmental focus, (2) working in depth, particularly with the transference and countertransference and thus accessing deep anxieties, and (3) adopting a stance that provides a containing therapeutic space, is thus supportive, and promotes possibilities for exploration. Though the model is not formulated primarily schematically in phases, the structure of the 16 sessions provides overlapping aspects of beginning, middle, and end.

In the beginning sessions, the transition from assessment to treatment is managed and its meaning explored, if this seems appropriate. The therapist will be sensitive to changes within the young person and the quality of material brought to the sessions. The focus on depth is encouraged through working with the relationship as it develops, using the countertransference as a powerful way of understanding emotionality and relatedness and working with the transference. In the middle sessions the young person may feel most securely "in" the therapy, and these sessions can be characterized by cooperative working on agreed aims, with the young person using the therapy as a space to bring what is on her/his mind. The process, pattern, and content may by now be relatively familiar, and anxieties may be more depressive in these sessions. However, this cannot be programmatic in practice, and the "middle" may be brief or may never arrive! Anxieties about engagement (beginning) and separation (ending) are always present to an extent, and the therapeutic work then consists of linking these anxieties to the therapeutic process through the transference. Anxieties about separation are inevitably more intense towards the end of the therapy, and it is important to contain these, to address the effects of the therapy and assess future options. One of the outcomes of time-limited therapy is the young person's engagement with the continuous project of her/himself, the development of her or his subjectivity and awareness of her or his emotionality. Reducing repeated or destructive relatedness to the self, gaining a more realistic view and greater openness to emotions in self and others, are key outcome factors for this form of therapy. These may lead to a wish for further therapy as an adolescent or "adult"; in these cases, it is the shift in the developmental process to a more depressive state of mind that constitutes a successful outcome for time-limited therapy and the greater integration of fears of loss of another and of separateness and separation.

Identification of a developmental focus for the intervention is crucial to this model of therapy. It is thought that through the therapeutic focus, for a time-limited period, on a significant area of developmental difficulty and/or disturbance, the adolescent/young adult patient will recover the capacity to meet developmental challenges and/or have this capacity strengthened. This focus involves attention placed on and intervention with maladaptive, stuck, regressive, or anti-developmental aspects of the self and also potentially developmentally supporting and sustaining aspects of the self. The focus will therefore be formulated in terms of the *presence* of anti-developmental factors that reduce the young person's capacity to engage with current life tasks and relationships, or the *absence* or weakness of resources that can promote growth and development. Establishing a focused exploration of the meaning of the young person's difficulties and symptoms within the process of adolescent development requires taking a view of the adolescent process as beginning with the adjustment to puberty and continuing through to the establishment of adult identity and roles. The developmentally based focus is articulated as being connected with one of the key underpinning aspects of adolescent development, applying the implications of the impact, meaning, and effects of puberty in separating from parental figures, taking ownership of the adult sexual body and of one's own thoughts and drives.

The developmental focus needs to fit closely the young persons' own account of themselves and their struggles and anxieties, to be related to the tasks and relationships they are involved with, and to encompass a sense of becoming, of encouraging curiosity about self and others. The therapist aims to tolerate—and enable the adolescent to also tolerate—the propensity to be up and down, excited, passionate, depressed, and, at times, the extremes of being both helplessly overwhelmed or irritatingly omnipotent. Moving between more negotiable and less available states of mind and requiring different responses from others is a significant part of this process.

Working with the impact of the time limit and ending means that therapists work under significant emotional pressure. There are particular tensions to manage—for example, to not hurry or to slow down change through recognizing developmental shifts. Osimo's (2003) ideas of recognizing "good" slowness or quickness references these aspects of time within the therapy. The capacity of the therapist to attain, in each session and also at different points in the session, the optimum therapeutic stance in relation to the young person requires considerable resources, flexibility, and attunement. Integral to this model of time-limited therapy is a weekly seminar group that discusses in detail the process of each therapeutic session, focuses on recognizing key trends in the transference and countertransference, and thus supports the therapist in being able to think about these and maintain a developmentally oriented focus. It is expected that as the young person moves rapidly between different states of mind and along a spectrum of ambivalence towards greater separateness and maturity, the therapist will need support in recognizing the way that the young person impacts on her; for these and other dynamics, the seminar group provides both support and the availability of a range of different perspectives. The seminar group fulfils the role of maintaining an overall view of the therapy and its boundary conditions, including the time limit. It is often important to include in the discussion the number of sessions that have taken place so far, or the number that remain. The seminar group takes responsibility for maintaining and reflecting on the developmental focus. This can help the therapist to feel more able to concentrate in the session on the issue of depth and the meaning of the therapeutic relationship as it develops.

Research on therapeutic interventions with young people

Research on psychodynamic/psychoanalytic therapeutic interventions with young people is limited by the impact of the service divide, through which adolescence is assimilated within child and adolescent services, on the one hand, and adult services for the over 18s on the other hand. Kronmuller, Stefini, Geiser-Elze, Hartmann, and Winkelmann (2010) detail the few studies for time-limited psychodynamic psychotherapy for children and adolescents; as they report, the studies that have been undertaken do show significant improvements for child and adolescents in psychodynamic/psychoanalytic treatments, including studies of the efficacy of disorder-specific treatments. However, it is difficult in these studies to separate out specifically the evaluation of treatments for adolescents. Baruch and Fearon (2002) undertook a follow-up study of young people over 16 seen at the Brandon Centre, London, based on analysis of their self-reports. In Sweden, Bjorn, Wennberg, Werbart, and Schubert (2006) studied young adults (age 18–25), comparing patient characteristics and outcomes. Overall, however, compared with studies of the behavioural therapies, there are very few studies that evaluate psychodynamic interventions for young people.

In developing a model of time-limited psychotherapy for young people, the aim has been to integrate the clinical service with the development of a strategy for evaluation. This has involved articulating and evaluating the approach through four areas: manualization, audit, study of process, and outcomes. The development of a manual aims to provide opportunities for replication and for testing the effectiveness through outcome study based on the focus of the model on developmental change. The manual articulates the aims and methods of the model, its core features and structure, and the role of the therapist (Lyon & Briggs, 2010).

The time-limited psychotherapy approach forms a small service in the Tavistock's Adolescent Department. There is an emphasis on a learning/teaching model, and this involves intensive support for trainees as well as staff, including the weekly seminar group and individual supervision. This restricts somewhat the capacity in the service for seeing large numbers of patients, but the fact that there are relatively few cases seen in the service also indicates resistance to referring cases for time-limited therapy when longer-term work is viewed as a preferable alternative. The limited evidence available for the effectiveness of psychodynamic psychotherapy suggests that ideally both time-limited and longer-term work should be available, and in this time-limited service it is helpful to work within an organizational framework where longer-term and more intensive approaches are available.

Time-limited therapy also provokes specific anxieties some therapists have with regard to setting time limits for young people, including providing a structured, boundaried setting for managing risks and disturbances; these can prevent appropriate and potentially beneficial use of a time-limited approach. We have gained a strong impression, which we are in the process of evidencing, that offering a time limit of, in our model, 16 sessions can have the effect of some young people receiving more therapy than when they are offered an open-ended treatment, from which they may drop out prematurely. Baruch's (2001) studies make a similar point. Moreover, the experiences young people have of current social contexts indicate that setting a time limit can provide a containing structure in an otherwise unstructured world.

Our audit data show that troubled young people do engage in therapy with this approach. Between September 2005 and July 2010, 31 cases—18 female and 13 male—ranging from 14 to 24 years in age have been offered time-limited therapy. Referral reasons evidence the complex psychosocial nature of the problems experienced by this group of young people; they present with a complex mixture of mental health difficulties—depression, anxiety, suicidal and self harming behaviour, interpersonal problems in family and relationships, and anxieties about social aspects of adolescent transitions. Of the 31 cases, 25 were assessed as suitable for time-limited therapy; 5 did not complete the assessment (having between 0 and 3 sessions). One case was assessed as not suitable for time-limited therapy. This young person did present a clear external time limit, but he also identified that he felt he had never had long enough in relationships with key people. The focus of his assessment therefore became how he could take up an open-ended therapy. Of the 25 young people who were offered time-limited therapy, 22 completed the treatment, and 10 came for a post-therapy review. Attendance rates were high for adolescents in therapy: 3 young people attended all 16 sessions, and 17 came for more than 10 sessions.

In applying the time-limited service, there is a strong commitment to relating measures of outcome to the developmental aims of the therapy and the therapeutic processes. Therefore, there is currently emphasis on examining processes and, through detailed descriptive accounts of therapies, identifying how cases fit—and refine—the model and how outcomes derived from the processes can be formulated. These outcomes are described developmentally, and relationally, with as much emphasis on supporting the young person's greater openness to reflection, including greater awareness of anxieties, as on reducing problematic behaviours. We think that often these two aspects are linked. The discussion of process and the qualities of outcomes can be illustrated here through describing a case in which we focus on interactions between adolescent patient and therapist. We present a young man in his mid-teens who feels threatened by a sense of failing to meet the developmental challenges of adolescence and whose vulnerability is experienced as a problem of maintaining his separateness from others—especially to be able to think his own thoughts and not fear collapse of himself or others. The case is described with reference to the key features of the model as described above.

Case example: Sam

Assessment

Sam's parents requested an assessment for psychotherapy when they became worried about his distress, agitation, and inability to sleep.

In the first assessment session, Sam, aged 15, soon became tearful: he said that he had "pressure from all sides" and that "everything is falling apart". He felt like he is failing at school and that "if he concentrates on one thing, then everything else crumbles". He described himself as having a breakdown, crying and not being able to sleep, fearing failure. He said that he tries his best, but nothing works and he fails, he doesn't meet his own and others' expectations. He was very worried about school work but also about not having a social life and not being able to communicate well with his parents. He said he had thoughts of suicide. After some exploration in the session the therapist asked him about his thoughts of coming to therapy, and he said he should be able to sort out his own problems by himself—thus, coming to therapy was another indicator of failure. He added, in an attempt to perhaps gain some distance from his distress, that some people had said that his problems "are just due to adolescence, and there may be some truth in this". At the end of this session it was agreed to meet on three further occasions to see whether he felt that therapy may be helpful.

In the seminar discussion of this session, the group wondered how extensive might be the sense of breakdown that Sam reported— whether it indicated an adolescent developmental crisis (Laufer & Laufer, 1984; Winnicott, 1961). Certainly he seemed to be very trapped by his persecuted and persecuting accusations of failure, and he appeared to be caught up in a very anxious and fearful sense of falling apart. Sam's parents had asked to be seen, and the group discussed the options: should the parents and Sam be seen together? Or should the parents be seen without Sam, and if so, at the same time, or at a different time? The importance of maintaining a separate space for Sam was thought to be the overriding priority at this point.

For the remaining assessment sessions, Sam made an effort to hold himself together and be less openly distressed. A key theme in the interactions in the session was the attempt Sam made to set a boundary between himself and his therapist, particularly, between what was on—or in—his mind and in his therapist's mind. He said that although his thoughts made complete sense to him, they might not make any sense to anyone else. He did not mind his parents knowing everything of what happened in his therapy, but he "would rather not speak about" things that are going on in his life. He wanted the therapist to ask questions but was anxious that the sessions might become an interrogation.

Thus Sam presented a particular dilemma for his therapy, which, when located in an adolescent developmental perspective, might be formulated thus: how can an adolescent, who has a fragile sense of his own independence, enter into therapy and allow himself to be dependent on a therapist? What can he share with the therapist? What is his, and what is the therapist's? Where to set a boundary? On the other side is an equally difficult question: what does the therapist need to know about, and what can be kept private? Perhaps above all other dilemmas in psychotherapy with adolescents, this is the one that most affects the technical aspects of the method, or, to put it another way, the adaptations to this issue make it different from psychotherapy with children, with adults, and, in fact, with young people at the late end of adolescence. The therapy thus needs to adapt to the adolescent's fragile sense of gathering within himself a sense of separateness from parental figures, his aloneness in the world, and the responsibility for his own thoughts and actions.

Sam's fear of failure and his current feeling that he *was* failing could be linked with this struggle to develop separateness from others—especially to be able to think his own thoughts and not fear collapse of himself or others. Thus the assessment identified a focus for Sam's therapy, stated as an adolescent developmental problem; it identified two key factors that indicated the potential benefits of a time-limited approach. In his social world Sam would be taking exams (GCSEs) in a few months, and this would to an extent test his capacity to be effective in the world or succumb to the fears of failure. In his internal world Sam seemed to need the structure of a therapeutic task that was manageable, rather than potentially overwhelming or, perhaps, entrapping. When he was offered 16 sessions, he said that this "seems just about right"

Therapy

Sam's therapy can be described through identifying three phases: In the first six sessions the focus was on difficulties of engagement. Sam was often late and, when in the room, he was cautious and withholding. In the middle sessions (6–10) there was a predominantly positive working alliance, followed, near the end of the therapy, by a tense, anxious, and often defiant and angry process of separating and ending.

In the first phase of therapy the therapist aimed to find moments of negotiability, or middle ground—a "space between yes and no" (Anthony, 1975) and also to attempt to introduce recognition of the delicate struggle for independence. For example, in the seminar group, Sam's therapist spoke of the discomfort of meeting him at reception and walking along the corridor with the sense of him dragging along five paces behind. The group thought that Sam's therapist could encourage him to check in at reception and make his own way to the room, and she could wait for him there. Tremulously he agreed to this, and with some self-consciousness he made his own way to the room, changed the sign on the door from "vacant" to "engaged", and shut the door very gently!

In the sessions, an issue arose about what he should tell his therapist and what he could withhold, or keep private. These discussions are helped in time-limited therapy by the therapist's low-key reminders of where they are in the time frame: linking this with external time-scales is important for the adolescent patient. Towards the end of the fifth session Sam's therapist mentioned, for example, that out of the 16 sessions they now had had 5. She added that this would take the end of the therapy into the exam period, and he might like to think whether they would need to take a break when the exams take place. She said it was his choice whether to continue with the weekly therapy or to take a break during the exam period. Sam was appreciative about having the choice and asked whether he could respond when he had a better idea of the actual dates of his exams.

The painfulness and delicacy of the predicament arising from the attempt to be more separate and individuated stirs sympathy in the therapist for the adolescent's struggles. It also requires that a sharp watch is kept on other trends, particularly those towards aggressiveness and hostility to the therapy and perversion of the attempts to help.

Sam's fear of feeling invaded by others had a corollary in his wish to invade, to get inside, and control others, particularly his parents. This aspect burst into the therapy when he was suspended from school for an incident involving breaking into an area reserved for staff use. He was reluctant to talk about this until the fear of further punishment receded. The perverse element lay in Sam maintaining he had achieved great success with organizing this break-in, and he would have felt worse if he had failed to do so. After some discussion of this, he said that he was quite worried about what he actually had the capacity to do: the phantasy of wishing to get inside the object was accompanied by the ability to actually do this. This new capacity for action is central to development in adolescence, as has been noted by, among others, Winnicott (1961), Hoxter (1964), and Anderson (1999). The acquisition of an adult sexual body means the adolescent has the physical means to put infantile phantasies into practice.

From the sixth session on, a more positive therapeutic alliance was evident. Sam opened up, talking about his fear of losing control and his fear of separation and having anxieties about his parents and his family; he was now looking at (and into) his parents, being anxious about seeing them as sexual adults. He was fearful of separating from them and feared that if one person left, then everything could crumble or fall apart.

In the seventh session Sam expressed discomfort with the idea of getting help from a teacher, and the therapist took up the transference. Sam responded by saying that with therapy he had made a choice to come, and he has realized that something happens in this room that doesn't happen elsewhere. He has found that talking in the way he talks here helps him to think clearly about things, so he has felt more comfortable about being open. He followed this by expressing regret about the therapy time he had missed, through being late, which he called "a real shame". He spoke rather movingly about having "an internal therapy room", which he imagines between his sessions.

In the middle session of time-limited therapy there is often a tremendous pressure on the therapist to relax the time frame and to change to an open-ended agreement. It may be that in some cases this is possible, but on the whole the risks outweigh the potential benefits, particularly as it will be difficult to overcome subsequent accusations of entrapment and the loss of credible authority through changing the contract. The challenge to the therapist in managing the ending of the therapy is a significant and demanding one, but the longer-term benefits for the adolescent patient are greater if the time frame can be sustained to facilitate the powerful emotional work of ending.

In the ending phase of Sam's therapy there was more overt defiance. In the fourteenth session, Sam arrived 10 minutes late and read a book throughout the session, not responding to any of the therapist's comments. The following week he was 30 minutes late, but he apologized for the previous week. When the therapist raised his defiance of her, he agreed with her interpretation that he had cut himself off from her in order to protect himself. He added that "I don't want to end, so I tried to break off from you. I want therapy to go on for ever and I want it to stop right now, so it doesn't drag out the pain." But, he added, as the therapy has been useful to him, he did not see the point in wasting the remaining sessions. This seemed to be a resourceful attempt to overcome his grievance and resentment and hold on to a hopeful good relation, to make the most of time available to him. In the remaining sessions he talked about feeling more positive in life and having a "different Sam to watch over the other Sam". The change in his development appeared to consist of a capacity both to be more open to others and also to regulate times when he did not have to be open, to be more in control of his thoughts and communication. He was thus able to confront his fears of failure, evidenced by being able to sit his exams.

Conclusion

This chapter has aimed to discuss the development of a time-limited psychodynamic psychotherapy for adolescents, emphasizing that this model is in the process of articulation and evaluation. Some strategies for undertaking this have included manualization and study of therapeutic processes. These precede evaluation of the effectiveness of the treatment method. This model is being developed as a relatively small service within a clinical unit specializing in working with young people. It applies an established approach to psychoanalytic therapy for young people that has been developed over time in the Tavistock's Adolescent Department and adapts this to provide a structured time-limited approach that may have wider applications in services working with young people with mental health difficulties.

The case example illustrates the processes of therapy and describes them in relation to the core characteristics of the therapeutic model. Sam is an example of a young person who can benefit from the experience of time-limited psychodynamic psychotherapy. In his mid-teens, he was fearful of failure—a fear of not being able to manage the adolescent developmental task of becoming more separate from his parental figures, particularly in the sense of feeling secure in having his own thoughts, in his own mind, separate from but also in communication with others.

The processes of assessment and therapy show the evolution of time-limited therapy based on a developmental focus, the role of the therapist and the seminar group in containing the emotional experiences of the therapist, and the young person's experiences of change. The case illustrates how young people make use of the containing function of the therapy to address difficulties they are having and to gain access to a more favourable developmental pathway.

At the core of the model is the view that through the therapeutic focus, for a time-limited period, on a significant area of developmental difficulty and/or disturbance, young people can recover the capacity to meet developmental challenges and/or have this capacity strengthened. This focus involves intervening with maladaptive, stuck, regressive, or anti-developmental aspects of the self. Similar importance is placed on containment to support aspects of the self that sustain development through adolescence.

Note

A version of this chapter was previously published in French as: Une psychothérapie psychodynamique développementale limitée dans le temps auprès d'adolescents et de jeunes adultes. Origines et applications. *Revue Adolescence, 29* (No. 2, 2011): 415–434.

References

Anderson, R. (1999). Introduction. In: D. Anastasopoulos, E. Laylou-Lignos, & M. Waddell, *Psychoanalytic Psychotherapy of the Severely Disturbed Adolescent*. London: Karnac.

Anderson, R., & Dartington, A. (1998). *Facing It Out: Clinical Perspectives on Adolescent Disturbance*. Tavistock Clinic Series. London: Duckworth.

Anthony, E. J. (1975). Between *yes* and *no*: The potentially neutral area where the adolescent and his therapist can meet. *Adolescent Psychiatry, 4*: 323–344.

Baruch, G. (Ed.) (2001). *Community-Based Psychotherapy with Young People: Evidence and Innovation in Practice*. Hove: Brunner-Routledge.

Baruch, G., & Fearon, P. (2002). The evaluation of mental health outcome at a community-based psychodynamic psychotherapy service for young people: A 12-month follow-up based on self-report data. *Psychology and Psychotherapy: Theory, Research and Practice, 75* (3): 261–278.

Bird, D. (1987). *The Adolescent Process and the Design of a Service for Adolescents.* Tavistock Clinic Paper No. 75. London: Tavistock and Portman NHS Foundation Trust Library.

Bird, D. (1989). *Adolescents and Negotiating Treatment.* Tavistock Clinic Paper No. 100. London: Tavistock and Portman NHS Foundation Trust Library.

Björn, P., Wennberg, P., Werbart, A., & Schubert, J. (2006). Young adults in psychoanalytic psychotherapy: Patient characteristics and therapy outcome. *Psychology and Psychotherapy: Theory, Research and Practice, 79* (1): 89–106.

Blos, P. (1962). *On Adolescence: A Psychoanalytic Interpretation.* New York: Free Press of Glencoe.

Briggs, S. (2008). *Working with Adolescents and Young Adults: A Contemporary Psychodynamic Approach.* Basingstoke: Palgrave Macmillan..

Briggs, S. (2009). Risks and opportunities in adolescence: Understanding adolescent mental health difficulties. *Journal of Social Work Practice, 23* (1): 49–64.

Charman, D. (Ed.) (2004). *Core Processes in Brief Psychodynamic Psychotherapy: Advancing Effective Practice.* Mahwah, NJ: Lawrence Erlbaum Associates.

Coren, A. (2009). *Short-Term Psychotherapy: A Psychodynamic Approach.* Basingstoke: Palgrave Macmillan.

Davanloo, H. (2000). *Intensive Short-Term Dynamic Psychotherapy: Selected Papers of Habib Davanloo.* Chichester: John Wiley.

Freud, S. (1918b [1914]). From the history of an infantile neurosis. *Standard Edition, 17:* 1–122.

Holmes, J. (1998). The changing aims of psychoanalytic psychotherapy: An integrative perspective, *International Journal of Psychoanalysis, 79:* 227–240.

Hoxter, S. (1964). The experience of puberty. *Journal of Child Psychotherapy, 1* (2): 13–26.

Jones, G. (2006). *The Thinking and Behaviour of Young Adults: Literature Review for the Social Exclusion Unit.* London: ODPM. Available at: http://wirrallearningpartnership.org/downloads/policies%2Cplans%20%2Cpublications

Kronmuller, K.-T., Stefini, A., Geiser-Elze, H., Hartmann, M., &

Winkelmann, K. (2010). The Heidelberg study of psychodynamic psychotherapy for children and adolescents. In: J. Tsiantis & J. Trowell (Eds.), *Assessing Change in Psychoanalytic Psychotherapy of Children and Adolescents: Today's Challenge*. London: Karnac.

Laufer, M., & Laufer, E. (1984). *Adolescence and Developmental Breakdown*. London: Karnac, 1995.

Lyon, L. (2004). Very brief psychoanalytically-based consultation work with young people. *British Journal of Psychotherapy, 21* (1): 30–35.

Lyon, L., & Briggs, S. (2010). *Manual for Time-Limited Psychodynamic Psychotherapy (for Adolescents and Young Adults) (TPP-A)*. Unpublished manuscript, Tavistock and Portman NHS Foundation Trust.

Malan, D. (1976). *The Frontier of Brief Psychotherapy*. New York: Plenum Press.

Malan, D., & Osimo, F. (1992). *Psychodynamics, Training and Outcome in Brief Psychotherapy*. London: Butterworth.

Mann, J. (1973). *Time-Limited Psychotherapy*. Cambridge, MA: Harvard University Press.

Osimo, F. (2003). *Experiential Short-term Dynamic Psychotherapy: A Manual*. Bloomington, IN: Authorhouse.

Patton, G., & Viner, R. (2007). Pubertal transitions in health. *Lancet, 369* (9567): 1130–1139.

Shefler, G. (1993). *Time-Limited Psychotherapy*. Jerusalem: The Hebrew University.

Shefler, G. (2000). Time limited psychotherapy with adolescents. *Journal of Psychotherapy Practice and Research, 9*: 88–99.

Waddell, M. (1998). *Inside Lives: Psychoanalysis and the Growth of the Personality*. Tavistock Clinic Series. London: Duckworth.

Waddell, M. (1999). Assessing adolescents: Process or procedure—the problems of thinking about thinking. *Psychoanalytic Inquiry, 19*: 215–228.

Waddell, M. (2002). The assessment of adolescents: Preconceptions and realizations. *Journal of Child Psychotherapy, 28* (3): 365–382.

Waddell, M. (2006). Narcissism: An adolescent disorder? *Journal of Child Psychotherapy, 32* (1): 21–34.

Walkerdine, V., Lucey, H., & Melody, J. (2001). *Growing Up Girl: Psychosocial Explorations of Gender and Class*. Chichester: Palgrave Macmillan.

Williams, A. H. (1978). Depression, deviation and acting-out in adolescence. *Journal of Adolescence, 1*: 309–317.

Winnicott, D. W. (1961). Adolescence: Struggling through the doldrums. In: *The Family and Individual Development*. London: Tavistock, 1965.

CHAPTER FOUR

The Young People's Consultation Services: a model of engagement

Linda Young & Frank Lowe

The adolescent process

As many writers, scientific and literary, have identified, adolescence is a turbulent period of profound change. The physical transformation initiated by the onset of puberty is but one of many, albeit one that is particularly striking and momentous. Any of us can observe how profound the change is when we look at a class of 11-year-olds, chronologically at the same age but, in terms of their physical development, very variable, ranging from those who are still pre-pubertal to those girls whose bodies are taking on a more adult, sexual form and who are beginning to menstruate, and boys who are growing taller, with voices breaking and increasing body hair. We know they will all need to negotiate these physical changes over the next few years, as we did ourselves in our own adolescence. Within this context of individual variability, puberty begins around the age of 10 and persists for approximately five years (Coleman & Hendry, 1999).

But there are other processes to be negotiated during this adolescent period. Along with the more overt physical changes prompted by increases in sexual and growth hormones are increases in sexual and aggressive drives, with accompanying and often highly charged and conflict-laden phantasies. The mental and emotional life of the adolescent takes on new dimensions that are challenging, exciting, and fearful. During puberty the girl comes to be able to carry a baby and the boy to impregnate a woman; both have the strength to cause physical damage to another in a way not possible during childhood years. These physical changes bestow a particular significance to sexual and aggressive phantasies, perhaps held unconsciously towards forbidden figures such as parents or siblings (see Blos, 1962, 1967; Klein, 1922; Waddell, 1998).

Puberty is a period of physical change that marks the onset of adolescence; adolescence itself is, however, characterized by a multitude of other changes and developmental tasks, which cover a much longer time span. The adolescent process broadly entails the shift from childhood relationships and contexts to those of adulthood. This period of transition requires becoming more independent of parents and family, developing a social, sexual, and work identity, and establishing close and committed adult sexual relationships. The psychological and emotional challenges of these developments are great and, it has been argued, increasingly so in contemporary Western society, with its complex opportunities and pressures relating to education, working life, and relationships (see, e.g., Furlong & Cartmel, 1997). While many young people have more educational opportunities than ever before, anxieties about getting employment are greater: more young people live at home for longer, which can be a source of helpful security, a base from which to grow, or a defensive retreat. At the same time, of course, social and family environments vary enormously for different adolescents. Some live in affluent parts of the country and enjoy a good education and material well-being; others live in poverty, in run-down, crime-ridden estates. There can be a sense of greater choice, but also greater uncertainty and unpredictability (see Briggs, 2008) and also greater inequality. These external contexts (levels of affluence, education, family environments) but also internal contexts (the nature of internalized early relationships, both good and bad) vary greatly between individuals. Both interact dialectically over time and will affect the potential for the individual adolescent to be able to manage the transition from being a child to being an adult. Globalization and technological progress provide new possibilities, but also new risks (Briggs, 2008; Graham, 2010).

Within this context of twenty-first-century society, a number of authors have pointed to a lengthening of the "adolescent" period.

Certainly it seems that some of the developmental tasks traditionally associated with adolescence now extend well into what tends generally to be thought of as young adulthood. Gluckman and Hanson (2006) write that the transition to adulthood tends to be completed around the age of 29/30, in contrast to the age of 23/24 some 50 years ago. Although they are specific in using marriage and parenthood as markers of the end of the transition period, other authors echo their conclusions (Graham, 2004; Patton & Viner, 2007).

While it would be inaccurate to suggest that all young people struggle with the transition, it is perhaps evident that adolescence is a period of particular physical, emotional, and social flux, which carries with it opportunities but also challenges and hazards. Indeed, it has long been noted that the adolescent/young adult period is the time when personality disorders tend to emerge, and there is a sharp increase in the number of those presenting with mental health problems. Many young adults with psychiatric disorders had had diagnosable difficulties younger in life—50% at 15 (Maughan, 2005). Additionally, there is evidence that levels of adolescent mental health difficulties are rising (Collishaw, Maughan, Goodman, & Pickles, 2004).

At the same time as figures indicate adolescence and young adulthood to be a period worthy of particular attention from mental health professionals, there is a lack of specialist provision (Lamb, Hall, Kelvin, & Van Beinum, 2008). Also, while some propose the benefit of intervention for mental health difficulties during these years, others advocate caution and leaving the way free for developmental processes to unfold in their own way, free from "interference". Not inconsistent with this can be an adolescent's own wish to be "left alone"—especially by adults, and perhaps especially also if those adults happen to be mental health professionals. The argument that this might be wise is not difficult to make, particularly when one considers that adolescence in itself could easily be judged by many a pathological process (Waddell, 2006). In addition, adolescents are often more drawn to action than to thought, to bullish independence rather than intimacy and the threat of dependency that talking to a therapist/psychologist/counsellor can entail. On the other hand, intervention in adolescence or young adulthood, at a time when the personality is in a state of flux, when there is greater fluidity and potential for change, could be seen as the most likely to succeed and to prevent more entrenched psychological difficulties from developing later.

The structure of services

Whatever one's view, in the United Kingdom the division of the structure of mental health services into Child and Adolescent (CAMHS) and Adult can make it difficult to provide age-appropriate help to young people seeking it for psychological or emotional difficulties (Singh et al., 2010). A number of recent Department of Health white papers have emphasized the importance of services bridging the gap between child and adult services and of providing services suitable for the adolescent/young adult age range—see the *National Service Framework for Mental Health* (DoH, 1999) and the *National Service Framework for Children, Young People and Maternity Services* (DoH, 2004)

The Young People's Counselling Service

The founders of the Young People's Counselling Service (YPCS)[1] thought it important to provide young people with the opportunity to talk to a professional about psychological and emotional difficulties. As touched on earlier, though, it is, of course, one thing to believe this as professionals and another to persuade others that this is the case— commissioners, for example, but also the young people themselves. Adolescents, striving to develop a sense of identity and autonomy, are notoriously reluctant to seek help, especially from adults. Fears of being psychically overwhelmed, of dependency, of capitulation to the adult world abound (Waddell, 1998). Seeking help for psychological ("mental") difficulties is particularly terrifying in the adolescent period, typified anyway by emotional and mental turbulence; secondarily, psychoanalysis can be one of the psychological sciences around which particular suspicions surface (Lowe, 2010). However, since its inception, it has always been the intention for the YPCS to offer a service that bridges the childhood and adult years by offering resources specifically to the adolescent/young adult age range (16–30). The intervention is brief in consisting of only four sessions; it is an intervention, but at the same time it embodies something of the "lack of interference" that is important to many young people. In this, the Service has always aimed to attract young people who might otherwise be unlikely to access any kind of mental health service—in other words, to make available something that may be acceptable to the most ambivalent and cautious of this already ambivalent group. Dartington (1995), writing about the YPCS, notes that as the Service is set up to be time-limited and to offer a contract of just four meetings, it tends to cater for a "particularly ambivalent" constituency. The term is not being used here in a derisory sense, but to capture something of the particularly powerful juxtaposition of the wish to know and the wish not to (Bion, 1962a, 1962b) that perhaps especially typifies those young people who take the step to ring up to make appointments to talk about themselves but do so within the particular context of the YPCS. Others may be motivated to contact the YPCS because there are few resources for this age group; some do not need or want longer-term therapy, some are "trying it out". Whatever the motivation, our expectation is that were it not for this particular context, some of the young people who approach us would certainly not be able to seek out psychological help for themselves, or at least not at that particular moment in their lives.

Background

Although our contemporary Young People's Consultation Services now include the Young Black People's Consultation Service (YBPCS) and a Parents' Service (which we shall not be discussing in detail in this chapter), the origins of these services are within the Young People's Counselling Service, established in 1961. The Service was set up with the intention of offering something specifically to adolescents and young people needing help to deal with any kind of problem (psychological, practical, medical); it was aimed at young people between the ages of 15 and 23 and was intended to offer prompt, easy-access help in a setting "independent of their world of authority" (see Lyon, 2004).

Contemporary contexts

Today the Service continues with the original endeavour to offer a space for thinking to those who might otherwise, for one reason or another, not access such help. With this in mind, ease of access, confidentiality, the brief, defined contract, and absence of contact with other professionals are crucial features of the Service. Ease of access is particularly facilitated by the self-referral nature of the Service and the fact that the young person only needs to ring our dedicated Service Coordinator to arrange the series of appointments. As mentioned, the Service offers four appointments—no more, no less, other than exceptionally. These are usually once weekly over four weeks, at the same time each week and for 50 minutes each time. A young person might not attend all four (replacing a missed session is an option, but it is certainly not automatic); some young people make use of a session through absence, which might subsequently be understood in a meaningful way.

The Service Coordinator acts as a gateway into the Service, gathering basic details (name, age, address, and a very brief outline of the reason for approaching the Service, checking GP details to ensure the young person falls within our NHS contract areas) and reiterating the nature of the Service (four sessions, finite, with a trained professional). This initial contact also allows some screening to help ensure that those who come to the Service are not obviously unlikely to be well served by such a very brief and very boundaried intervention; in such cases, the help offered will be in this telephone call, by the Service Coordinator providing information on alternative, more appropriate sources of help. The Service is staffed by qualified, experienced mental health professionals, many of whom are gaining further experience in working within a very brief consultation model and/or with the particular age range served by the YPCS. All therapists within the Service attend a weekly seminar group, taken by one of the Adolescent Department senior staff experienced in working within the Service. In this group, material from sessions is presented in detail, the varying reactions and thoughts of individual group members typically providing rich sources of further understanding about the client.

The defined contract of four sessions, clearly stipulated at the outset, is intended to allow young people to engage with us when they may be fearful of committing to anything lengthier. Similarly, we are clear in maintaining the boundary around the four sessions and making no links with parents or other professionals, other than when absolutely necessary—which happens rarely and is typically due to risk concerns of some kind. We do not make referrals on after the four sessions; information may be given about sources of further help, but the responsibility for taking this further is left clearly with the young person. Typical adolescent fears of becoming overwhelmed, overdependent, regarded as "mad", or entangled in some fearful adult mental health context are potentially allayed by these features of the Service.

The consultation:
a triangular space

The sessions aim to encourage a process of self-discovery rather than dependency. Not fostering a dependent relationship with the therapist makes sense, of course, in such a time-limited therapeutic encounter but also acknowledges the importance of recognizing, supporting, or perhaps contributing to the development of qualities of independence and self-determination in late adolescents/young adults. While not exclusively one or the other, the emphasis of the YPCS encounter is on knowing more about rather than working through difficulties. Sometimes this can mean an entirely different conceptualization of the problem—the 18-year-olds who come with exam-related stress, who begin to know more about their anxiety about leaving home (which may not be possible, they report, if they do not pass their exams), and that this anxiety is linked with an early history of loss in a significant relationship. The therapist is thinking and talking with the young person *about* their presenting difficulties. Rather than a dyad (therapist and client) in the consulting room, one might conceptualize the encounter as a triad, with the counsellor consulting to the "healthy" part of the client about the "troubled" part of themselves.

The notion of different elements of the personality, with splits between more healthy and more disturbed parts of the self, is well represented in the analytic literature (see, e.g., Bion, 1967; Rosenfeld, 1987; Steiner, 1986). Defensive splitting allows what are usually conflicting thoughts, feelings, or aspects of the self to be kept apart, and protected (a healthy part of the self protected from being overwhelmed by madness, for example). Bion writes about different parts of the personality, functioning more or less well in relation to reality, in his description of psychotic and non-psychotic parts of the self (Bion, 1967). The young people seen in the YPCS are not psychotic in the psychiatric sense, but they are bringing a problem that they cannot solve. One might conceptualize the act of seeking help as done by a healthy part of the personality that seeks assistance for a troubled part. Of course, seeking help is not always such a straightforward act, nor does it necessarily have such a meaning, but we think that within the YPCS it is helpful to think of one's task as one where the endeavour is to engage the healthy part of the personality in thinking about the disturbed or distressed part. This notion of a healthy, observing component of the ego being present and able to know about more disturbed aspects was described as far back as Freud (1940e [1938]).

Rather than directly address and work with the troubled part of the personality (for example, in the transference), one might observe this part present in the room but seek to work with the functioning and observing aspects of the ego to think about the problem. So the therapist might well notice and reflect on aspects of the transference relationship, as well as the way the young person relates to the Service itself (to the first, middle, and ending "phases"—that is, the first session, the second and third sessions, and then the fourth, final session: why are they coming now?) but then use these observations to talk to the young person about his or her conflicts and anxieties and ways of relating rather than taking it up directly in relation to the therapist. Talking to the client about the transference to the therapist is generally avoided in order to titrate the emotional intensity of this relationship when it is soon to come to an end and in order to engage the young person in being responsible for thinking about him/herself. Dependency on the process of thinking rather than on the therapist is encouraged (see Dartington, 1995; Lyon, 2004; Oliver-Bellasis, 1998).

There is debate about the concept of *triangular space* (Meissner, 2006), but it is perhaps helpful to think of the YPCS encounter in this way—as a *triangular space* (client, therapist, problem) in which thinking may be able to flourish. Ron Britton makes reference to this in writing about psychoanalytic work and reflecting on the internal process that allowed the analyst to comment on the patient (Britton, 2004). Britton's notion conceptualizes the triangular space in oedipal terms—parents in interaction in relation to the child. In the conceptualization offered here, the young person is part of a couple, in consultation with the YPCS therapist about his or her own (the client's) troubled self. The client is both parenting and dependent, in a way that captures something of the developmental "in-betweenness" of the late adolescent/young adult state. Indeed, to reflect this, latterly the name of the YPCS has been changed to Young People's Consultation (rather than Counselling) Service.

The seminar group

The group process in the weekly supervision seminar held for all YPCS therapists (with around 6 therapists in each) is an important facet of the overall process. This is perhaps because of working so briefly; material can more readily be digested in a group, where responses to the material can be (unconsciously) shared between participants—for example, one might respond maternally to the same material that causes another to feel angry; both might be relevant to understanding. The countertransference experience of the consultation, both by the therapist in the room with the client and with the group in hearing the material of the session subsequently presented, regularly helps to clarify where the issues and anxieties lie. The group seminar offers another triangular space for thinking (group members, therapist, material) that parallels that between client, therapist, and the client's difficulties. The seminars are usually 90 minutes, but two or three clients may be discussed within that time. While it is important that material is brought and discussed in detail, the limited time available (possibly only 30 minutes per client presentation) also parallels the limited time of the four session contract and fosters thinking that focuses on extracting and articulating key themes, as needs to happen in the YPCS consultation itself, where one hopes to be able to focus on central anxieties that the client is currently experiencing, to name them and so make them available for thought (Dartington, 1995).

The seminar group also has the important function to contain some of the anxieties that can be raised by the particular challenges of such very brief work; it can allow us to think about all aspects brought by our clients—and to think through when and how and if to talk about them in the sessions. Anxieties can be stirred, for example, by the fact that we know very little about our clients before we see them—there are no formal referral letters—and with only four sessions may worry about what can be achieved; ending can be painful for the therapist as well as the client. Guilt about ending at a moment when something feels as though it has just begun can be hard to tolerate, although often such feelings take on particular qualities with particular clients and are a further source of information and understanding about the young person. Of course it is always important to distinguish when a "countertransference" reaction tells us more about the young person, as opposed to more about our own personalities and struggles (see also Lemma, 2003).

The aim of the consultation is to help put into words core issues and anxieties, identifying things that up to that point may have been hidden or obscured by confusion. As described, the consultation does not aim to work through the young person's difficulties, but to name them in a way that may not have hitherto happened; for some this is enough in itself. For others it is not, but as the YPCS is regarded very much as a piece of work in its own right, *not* an assessment for psychotherapy, the question of more therapy or counselling is generally not raised by the therapist unless the client raises it him/herself.

Clinical example

Maria, aged 22, had not had any previous therapy or counselling when she rang the YPCS and told our Service Coordinator that she was prompted to contact the Service because she was feeling anxious and depressed. In elaborating on this, she added that when was out in bright sunlight, she "saw the light and saw everything differently" and then felt frightened that she was going to have a panic attack. Having met her, the therapist described Maria as physically slight, dark-haired, pale-skinned, dressed all in black with just a splash of colour in a scarf; although wearing no make-up, she appeared rather chic. The overall impression was of a mixture of sophistication and innocence, with something very young about her appearance and manner.

In the first session Maria linked her first spell of anxiety with taking ecstasy; she had been taking it in the two years prior to her first attack of anxiety, around once every two weeks, maybe once monthly. In the last 18 months, since the first episode of feeling so anxious, she had not taken any drugs. Maria was tearful in the session, speaking of her fear that she was going crazy and describing in more detail how, particularly in bright daylight, things became so vivid, everything looked so different; she felt bombarded with light and colour and images.

In the subsequent seminar group, the therapist spoke of herself feeling rather confused and anxious, and the members of the group echoed this, being uncertain what to make of the experiences Maria had described—some thought that Maria's experiences might be drug-related, others that this may be the beginnings of a psychotic illness, and yet others that she just appeared very young and in need of reassurance. The seminar leader felt herself bombarded and overwhelmed and feeling alone responsible for understanding the material. This left her wondering whether Maria's experience was of being faced with experiences that had proved overwhelming, and in the absence of any figure that could really help her to understand and manage them.

> As the session continued, Maria spoke about the second occasion when she had been severely affected by anxiety, 12 months previously. She had been returning to England from a visit to her home country (which, she clarified, was France) when, mid-flight, the plane was rocked by serious turbulence, and she was gripped by a crippling fear that it was going to crash. The therapist said to Maria that she was speaking of a fear that some disaster was about to befall her—but this might be something other than the plane literally crashing, maybe more to do with something else collapsing, crashing down in her or in her life; she seemed terrified that something catastrophic was going to happen. Maria burst into tears then in the session and related that during the visit to France she had seen her father for the first time in four years, and he had told her that he had been addicted to cocaine for the last two years. Maria also spoke of the fact that her parents were divorced and that she did not feel she could talk with her mother about the news of her father's addiction. Indeed, it appeared that Maria's experience was of being left alone with rather frightening and difficult things—also things about people whom she might expect to be looking after her.

The therapist reported to the seminar group that she was struck that four years had passed without contact between Maria and her father, and that she had asked Maria about this. The seminar group were concerned about such a direct question, particularly when the therapist went on to report that, on being asked about it, Maria had become manifestly panicky in the room, saying that she felt dizzy and unwell and could not talk.

> After a few moments, with her head in her hands and breathing deeply, Maria looked up and said that she now felt okay, but had been feeling as she did when in the light: overwhelmed and anxious.

The therapist described being concerned in the session about the impact the comment seemed to have had on Maria, and the group debated the timeliness of the intervention, and whether it was wise to have made it at all. However, there was also discussion of the session as an opportunity to address these issues. In the group, the conflict about looking and seeing versus turning a blind eye (Steiner, 1990) was very evident.

> Returning to the second session, the therapist took this up with Maria in terms of part of her wanting to use the sessions to see things more clearly, but another part of her being very frightened of doing that. Maria then told the therapist that the period of no contact with her father had followed an argument about money. The therapist was very struck by the extent to which they had been able to cut off from each other—and thereby presumably from their feelings about each other—for such a long time. When the therapist queried this, Maria said that she "just didn't think about it", that she was busy with other things. The therapist wondered whether Maria's making contact again with her father resulted in a sudden dissolution, a sudden collapse of her "cut-off" state, in a way that was quite devastating. She commented that she thought Maria was very anxious now about the state her father was in, perhaps particularly after being out of contact with him for so long (she thought perhaps suddenly leaving Maria besieged with guilt, with no one available to help her with it).

Maria went on to describe more details about her parents' divorce. Her parents had separated when she was 13 years old. Although subsequently they tried to repair their relationship, it had broken down again, resulting in divorce. Maria said that she had been surprised when her parents first separated; she had not had any sense that this was about to happen, but she had not been upset. The therapist was struck by how cut-off Maria seemed, commenting that it was a big thing to have happened in her life. More thoughtfully, Maria then remarked that she did not know why she was not upset. Perhaps because she was busy enjoying life at the time, going out with friends.

Maria then spoke of her father always having been more like a friend than a parent. Her mother, she said, had set the rules and boundaries in their home; she was conservative, concerned with budgeting, finances, keeping the household going. Father had been rather the opposite, drinking, smoking drugs, staying out late and not letting anyone know where he was. These descriptions added to her story about her father's anger when she had asked him for money: Maria's mother had often asked for money from father, concerned herself about budgeting carefully, while he did not want to think about it at all. Nor did he, Maria described, want to think about anything difficult or demanding; rather than address it, he would, instead, drink or go out in order to blot out whatever the problem was. It also then seemed as though her father's cocaine addiction was not particularly out of character. The therapist suggested to Maria that she may feel conflict in herself between identifying with her mother's more careful and conservative attitude and her father's more liberal one. Maria replied that she used to be more like her father, but in the last year and a half or so had become more like her mother. The therapist pointed out that this was also the period in which she had become more anxious and unwell, and she wondered whether this related to the loss of a particular way of managing difficulties, which had been her father's way—blotting out in various ways anything troubling. Maria commented that she did indeed now worry about all sorts of things in a way she never had.

After this session, the seminar group felt that they were overall beginning to piece together a picture of Maria and her life, but wondered how much Maria—as opposed to the therapist and the group—had been able to take any of this in and make use of it to understand herself and her difficulties a little more.

Then, somewhat surprisingly to the group, Maria began the third session by saying that she had been thinking about what had been talked about last time, and particularly how much she had changed, and how it was different from being like her father. In the last year and a half she had been preoccupied by worries; in the past she had been hard, cut off, but now she had lost that and in a way regretted it. The therapist commented that Maria had maybe tried to cut off from much that could cause her anxiety and other troubling feelings, and that when this did not work, she found herself confronted in a very unsettling way with all that had been pushed away—she suddenly saw the turbulence around and inside herself and then started to panic (the therapist was here thinking about the earlier description Maria gave of being caught in turbulence during her plane flight). Maria replied that sometimes she wondered whether something had upset her or not; she did not know, she added quietly: "I think I got very good at cutting off." In spite of her ambivalence about knowing more about herself, Maria did now seem to be discovering something of her way of trying to deal with difficulties—which perhaps had not been contained for her by her mother, who became very anxious, or by her father, who couldn't bear to know. It seemed possible that at the point in her life when she was literally separating from her home country and her closer proximity to her parents and beginning more clearly the transition into adult life, conflicts over identity and unresolved difficulties connected with this and with loss broke through her existing defensive organization, leaving Maria flooded on occasion with anxiety and panic.

Maria was 15 minutes late for the last of the four sessions, having previously always been on time. She arrived breathless, explaining that she had forgotten the time and then had to rush to get to the session but could not then avoid being late. Maria then spoke of not feeling very well in the last week, feeling more anxious again, although not experiencing the panic that had led her to seek help in the first place: that seemed to have settled. She commented that she did not know why she had been feeling badly in the last week, or indeed why she had been experiencing panic and anxiety in the first place; she knew that links had been made in the sessions with some of her experiences, and the links made sense, but they were such little things. The therapist questioned whether what Maria had discussed were such little things. Maria replied that she tried not to get upset and always tried to distract herself, including over the last several days. The therapist commented that perhaps she was trying to distract herself from feelings about this being the last of the four sessions, which was also not such a little thing. The therapist wondered whether this had contributed to Maria being late, it being difficult to come for the last time. Maria said that she was not aware of being upset, but perhaps she was; it left her wondering about whether to take things further or not, and how. The therapist commented that the "how" could be answered by sending her some information on further sources of therapy, but whether or not to do it was perhaps the dilemma Maria felt left with—part of her wanted to, and part of her did not.

In the group, there were mixed opinions about whether Maria was likely to pursue further help; this was speculative—we did not find out whether she had or not. It is often one of the difficulties of the YPCS work that we are left not knowing what happened next. At the same time, there is perhaps some relief for us too as counsellors in not needing to know, having offered four sessions but not being in a position to offer more.

The Young Black People's Consultation Service

While the origins of the YPCS were in the context of recognizing a lack of facilities for young people, in the early 2000s the lack of service provision that specifically embraced questions of race and culture led to the establishment of the Young Black People's Consultation Service. The initial aim of the Young People's Consultation Service to allow access to a population who might otherwise not engage with mental health services—the population of adolescents/young adults—was strongly in evidence in this later endeavour to try to make psychological therapies more accessible to young black people and their families. The new Service adopted key aspects of the YPCS model, in being also very brief (typically four sessions), psychoanalytically informed (noting the transference and drawing on the countertransference), and, crucially, embodying the kind of informality and lack of interference at the heart of the intervention. This was evidenced in the referral process—again allowing self-referral, without needing GP involvement—and in the nature of the process as one that is essentially about sitting and thinking together about the issues, rather than one with a defined aim like an assessment *for* something else.

At the same time, the original intent to be responsive to perceived need—originally that of the young adult population—informed the evolution of the YBPCS and led to significant differences, which were incorporated, with the aim of being responsive to some particular issues significant to working with young black people.

The YBPCS therefore accepts referrals from parents and community bodies, particularly schools. It also aims to provide consultations in settings that young black people regard as comfortable and accessible—such as schools, community centres, and youth clubs. The YBPCS is, also, open to young black people from the age of 14, rather than 16. This is because of the high numbers of young black people aged 14/15 being excluded from local schools for "emotional and behavioural problems" who do not access psychological therapies prior to or after exclusion. Indeed, black and "other black" students are three times more likely to be excluded from schools in England and Wales than are white students (Ofsted, 2008). The YBPCS accepts self-referrals, but also referrals from parents, carers, and professionals, not only because we recognize that younger adolescents—the 14–15-year-olds—are less likely to self-refer, but also because many young black people, especially, and particularly those most disaffected, are unlikely to know about or be willing to initiate contact with mental health services (see SCMH, 2006). In line with this, consultations are also provided to parents, carers, and professionals if the young person about whom they are concerned refuses to engage with the Service. In this respect, the YBPCS incorporates a second service, which has evolved from the YPCS: the Parents' Consultation Service—a service offering four sessions to self-referring parents who want to talk about the difficulties of their adolescent (aged 14–25) where the young person is not him/herself willing to engage with services.

The intention of all these services is to work with the adolescent process, but also with the adolescent social and cultural context. For the YBPCS, the adaptations mentioned above are part of the attempt to do this. Seventy percent of BME (black and minority ethnic) groups live in the 88 most deprived areas in Britain, compared with 40% of whites (SEU, 2000); young black people are more likely to be poor than are white children; and they are overrepresented in populations with greater mental health needs, such as children excluded from school, children in public care, and young offenders (BMA, 2003; SEU, 2000). Therefore, black adolescents living in Britain have to struggle to establish a positive and cohesive identity, not only because of their individual characteristics and family experience, but also because of the nature of the dominant social and cultural context, which includes racism and cultural prejudice. These pressures can lead some young black people to deny or reject their culture or to feel that it is inferior, and others to become alienated from mainstream society. The mental stress and vulnerability of young black people in the United Kingdom appear to be further exacerbated by difficulties in accessing appropriate supportive mental health services. Black people, particularly those from African, African Caribbean, and mixed-parentage communities, are also reluctant to seek help for psychological and emotional difficulties and are more likely to come to the attention of mental health services involuntarily through sectioning under the Mental Health Act (MIND, 1988). One study found that a young black person living in London is four times more likely to be an inpatient in a psychiatric ward than is a young white person (SCMH, 2006). The YBPCS is very mindful of this context and regards the ability to understand it and work with black people's suspiciousness of mental health services as important requirements in its work.

Clinical example

Ade, aged 14, was referred by his GP to the YBPCS because he had been excluded from school, was refusing to attend the Pupil Referral Unit (PRU) he had been referred to, and had become withdrawn at home. Ade was an only child who had been brought up largely by his mother. His mother was from Africa and his father from the Caribbean, and they had a very unstable relationship, with father moving in and out of the family home several times from the time Ade was about 2 years old. Ade had a history of emotional and behavioural difficulties dating back to primary school and had been referred several times to the local CAMHS. Although he and his mother attended a few appointments together, they had never fully engaged with the local CAMHS.

Ade's parents were very worried because they thought that he was showing signs of depression and anxiety but was refusing to see a mental health professional. His mother, having heard about the YBPCS from a friend, referred the family to the Service. Ade, however, refused to attend, and we agreed to offer four consultation appointments to his parents to think about the situation together and to explore what might be helpful.

Both parents were punctual for the first appointment. They appeared to be very different in a number of ways: the mother,

Shola, was a secretary in the City; she had a quiet professional demeanour but seemed quite sad and worried. Leroy, Ade's father, was a car mechanic. He was very muscular, had a strong physical presence, and came across as confident and relaxed. They spoke openly about Ade and their history as parents. They had been living together for a few years when Shola became pregnant with Ade. Their relationship broke down when Shola was 6 months pregnant, and as a result Leroy moved out before Ade was born. He did, however, try to keep in touch with Ade as much as possible and, of course, saw much more of him during the periods he lived with them. On reflection, he acknowledged that he had been an absent father for much of Ade's childhood, and he felt guilty about that.

They both described Ade as getting into lots of fights in primary school, often because he was provoked by peers or picked on by teachers. His behaviour had improved in secondary school and had been stable during the past year. But he was permanently excluded because a male teacher had not believed him when he said he had not done his homework due to illness. Ade's reaction led to staff perceiving him as having an "anger management problem" and that this might be partly related to him feeling neglected by his father. In the consultation, the therapist wondered about whether and how Ade expressed vulnerable feelings; this led to the parents remarking on what they considered some puzzling things about him, which were times when he had shown great anxiety in social situations and become withdrawn. The therapist then asked Shola how she had been affected by the break-up of the relationship with Leroy. This led to a moving account of the difficulties and her sadness, and then to an acknowledgement that the current situation may be confusing and arousing for Ade, as Leroy had started living with them again about two months before Ade's exclusion from school.

Prior to the second appointment, the therapist received a call from Leroy stating that Shola was unable to attend the appointment, and he wondered whether he could attend on his own. The therapist confirmed that it was important to see them both. At the second appointment Ade's father had great deal to say. It was as if the first appointment had brought up a lot of memories and feelings. He said that he knew what it was like to be like Ade.

He had had a very difficult childhood, including being bullied and isolated at school and not having a good relationship with his father. Mother had seemed sad and had been relatively quiet in the session. Eventually she stated that she was sad because a close uncle had died, and that she hadn't heard Leroy speak like this before. In fact, she was sad that they didn't really speak at all. She hadn't really ever spoken to him about the extent of her sadness when he had left before Ade was born. By the end of the session they both acknowledged how little they spoke about their deep feelings, how remarkably similar Ade was to Leroy, and how Shola's sadness and anger about Leroy's neglect of her was unexpressed.

By the third appointment, Shola reported that during the past three weeks Ade had shown gradual but growing interest in the consultation. The therapist suggested that she encourage him to come to an appointment. At the end of the fourth and last appointment with his parents, Shola reported that Ade had said that he would like to come to an appointment, but not with his parents. The therapist offered Ade an appointment a few weeks after concluding the consultation with the parents. In reviewing the consultation, the parents stated that the sessions had helped them enormously. They had learnt that probably for most of Ade's childhood they had not listened to him enough. They recognized that he was very anxious about going to school, and they had stopped trying to force him to attend the PRU and had, instead, obtained some home tuition for him. As a result he was much more relaxed and seemed a little happier. His tutor also thought he had a real flair for writing and was encouraging him to write short stories. Shola and Leroy thought that they needed to sort out their unstable and unclear relationship because they had never given sufficient thought to how it affected Ade but, more importantly, to what it meant really and where it was going. They found the opportunity to talk and think about these things very helpful and went away convinced that they wanted to continue to come to talk about their relationship and their parenting of Ade. They were referred to the Parents' Service. Ade attended his consultation appointment and went on from there to start open-ended psychotherapy within the Tavistock Adolescent Department.

Conclusion

Adolescents' reluctance and conflict about seeking help, especially with their most personal and private problems, is probably familiar to the majority of professionals who work with this age group. Reluctance and conflict can be compounded for young people from black and minority ethnic communities because of cultural factors and, perhaps, the inaccessibility of mental health services. The consultation model described is not only a way of making help with mental health problems easier to access for many young people, it is also a model of engaging adolescents and young adults therapeutically without threatening their much-valued sense of independence. Recently, outcome data have shown the effectiveness of the consultation (see Searle, Lyon, Young, Wiseman, & Foster-Davis, 2011).

Therapeutic consultations are interventions in their own right, and for some young people they can also be a helpful bridge to longer-term help for serious problems. In either case, we hope to have illustrated that although brief, these interventions can be of significant—and, in some cases, long-standing—therapeutic power.

Note

1. The YPCS, originally known as "The Young People's Counselling Service", is now known as the "The Young People's Consultation Service".

References

Bion, W. R. (1962a). *Learning from Experience*. London: Karnac, 1984.
Bion, W. R. (1962b). A theory of thinking. *International Journal of Psycho-analysis, 43*: 306–10. Also in: *Second Thoughts*. London: Karnac, 1984.
Bion, W. R. (1967). *Second Thoughts*. London: Karnac, 1984.
Blos, P. (1962). *On Adolescence: A Psychoanalytic Interpretation*. New York: Free Press of Glencoe.
Blos, P. (1967). The second individuation process of adolescence, *Psychoanalytic Study of the Child, 22*: 162–186.
BMA (2003). *Adolescent Mental Health*. London: British Medical Association.

Briggs, S. (2008). *Working with Adolescents and Young Adults: A Contemporary Psychodynamic Approach.* Basingstoke: Palgrave Macmillan.

Britton, R. (2004). Narcissistic disorders in clinical practice. *Journal of Analytical Psychology, 49* (4): 477–490.

Coleman, J., & Hendry, L. (1999). *The Nature of Adolescence* (3rd edition). London: Routledge.

Collishaw, S., Maughan, B., Goodman, R., & Pickles, A. (2004). Time trends in adolescent mental health. *Journal of Child Psychology and Psychiatry, 45* (8): 1350–1362.

Dartington, A. (1995). Very brief psychodynamic counselling with young people. *Psychodynamic Counselling, 1* (2).

DoH (1999). *National Service Framework for Mental Health: Modern Standards and Service Models.* London: Department of Health.

DoH (2004). *National Service Framework for Children, Young People and Maternity Services: The Mental Health and Psychological Well-Being of Children and Young People.* London: Department of Health/HMSO.

Freud, S. (1940e [1938]). Splitting of the ego in the process of defence. *Standard Edition,* 23: 271–278.

Furlong, A., & Cartmel, F. (1997). *Young People and Social Change: Individualization and Risk in Modern Society.* Buckingham: Open University Press.

Gluckman, P., & Hanson, M. (2006). Evolution, development and timing of puberty. *Trends in Endocrinology and Metabolism, 17:* 7–12.

Graham, P. (2004). *The End of Adolescence.* Oxford: Oxford University Press.

Graham, R. (2010). Use of technology and addiction to it. *Government Gazette,* April/May.

Klein, M. (1922). Inhibitions and difficulties at puberty. In: *Love, Guilt and Reparation and Other Works* (pp. 54–58). London: Hogarth Press, 1975.

Lamb, C., Hall, D., Kelvin, R., & Van Beinum, M. (2008). *Working at the CAMHS/Adult Interface: Good Practice Guidance for the Provision of Psychiatric Services to Adolescents/Young Adults.* A joint paper from the interfaculty working group of the Child and Adolescent Faculty and the General and Community Faculty of the Royal College of Psychiatrists. Available at: www.rcpsych.ac.uk/pdf/Transition_2008.pdf

Lemma, A. (2003). *Introduction to the Practice of Psychoanalytic Psychotherapy.* Chichester: John Wiley.

Lowe, F. (2010). Working with ambivalence, making psychotherapy more accessible for young black people. In: A. Lemma & M. Patrick (Eds.), *Off the Couch: Contemporary Psychoanalytic Applications.* London: Routledge.

Lyon, L. (2004). Very brief psychoanalytically-based consultation work with young people. *British Journal of Psychotherapy, 21* (1): 30–35.

Maughan, B. (2005). Continuities between childhood and adult life. *British Journal of Psychiatry, 187*: 301–333.

Meissner, W. (2006). The therapeutic alliance: A proteus in disguise. *Psychotherapy—Research, Practice and Training, 3* (3): 264–270.

MIND (1988). *The Mental Health of the African and Caribbean Community in Britain. Factsheet.* London: MIND Publications.

Ofsted (2008). *Reducing Exclusions of Black Pupils from Secondary Schools: Examples of Good Practice.* Reference No. 070240. Manchester: Ofsted.

Oliver-Bellasis, E. (1998). Is anyone there? The work of the Young People's Counselling Service. In: R. Anderson & A. Dartington (Eds.), *Facing It Out: Clinical Perspectives on Adolescent Disturbance.* London: Duckworth.

Patton, G., & Viner, R. (2007). Pubertal transitions in health. *Lancet, 369* (9567): 1130–1139.

Rosenfeld, H. (1987). *Impasse and Interpretation.* London: Tavistock Publications.

SCMH (2006). *The Costs of Race Inequality.* Policy Paper 6. London: Sainsbury Centre for Mental Health. Available at www.centreformentalhealth .org.uk/pdfs/costs_of_race_inequality_policy_paper_6.pdf

Searle, L., Lyon, L., Young, L., Wiseman, M., & Foster-Davis, B. (2011). The Young People's Consultation Service: An evaluation of a consultation model of very brief psychotherapy. *British Journal of Psychotherapy, 27* (1): 56–78.

SEU (2000). *Minority Ethnic Issues in Social Exclusion and Neighbourhood Renewal.* London: Social Exclusion Unit/Cabinet Office.

Singh, S., Paul, M., Ford, T., Kramer, T., McLaren, S., Howish, K., et al. (2010). Process, outcome and experience of transition from child to adult mental health care: Multiperspective study. *British Journal of Psychiatry, 197*: 205–212.

Steiner, J. (1986). *Psychotic and Non-Psychotic Parts of the Personality in Borderline States.* London: Tavistock Clinic.

Steiner, J. (1990). The retreat from truth to omnipotence in Sophocles' *Oedipus at Colonus. International Journal of Psychoanalysis, 17*: 227–235.

Waddell, M. (1998). *Inside Lives: Psychoanalysis and the Growth of the Personality.* Tavistock Clinic Series. London: Duckworth.

Waddell, M. (2006). Narcissism: An adolescent disorder? *Journal of Child Psychotherapy, 32* (1): 21–34.

CHAPTER FIVE

Complexity in primary care

Brian Rock & Anca Carrington

In recent years there has been an unprecedented investment in mental health within primary care and through the Improving Access to Psychological Therapies (IAPT) programme. This has led to the establishment of services primarily offering cognitive behavioural therapy to those people with common mental health problems—that is, mild to moderate anxiety and depression. Lord Layard, the architect of the IAPT programme, made a compelling financial case for such investment—around £173 million in the first three years—because he was able to demonstrate how such provision would enable those people unable to work and requiring incapacity benefit to return to work, thereby becoming more productive in society and more fulfilled in their lives.

IAPT has done what it says on the tin, so to speak, enabling thousands of people to access psychological help who would have not been able to meet the threshold criteria for secondary care services. If you imagine the stepped care model as a pyramid, with the more complex, specialist services/interventions provided closer to the apex, then IAPT services have strengthened the foundation in primary care and aimed to improve links with secondary/tertiary services.

Notwithstanding its obvious benefits, there are also concerns about IAPT. Chiefly, these include: the extent to which the role of GPs, especially in relation to the management and treatment of depression, has been overlooked, even diminished, in the original Layard report (Elder, 2009); the almost exclusive focus on the provision of one therapeutic modality, though this is now shifting with the inclusion of other evidence-based approaches; and the reliance on the least qualified or least experienced clinicians for triage and assessment, especially when this involves contact with patients who fall outside the mild–moderate spectrum.

With the expected budgetary cuts set out in the government's spending review, especially in areas such as welfare and the consequent savings required in mental health provision, along with the anticipated raising of the referral threshold into secondary care, this is likely to increase the demand on the primary care system—the care system that is the focus of this chapter.

We begin this chapter by setting out a picture of the realities of primary care with an emphasis on the role of the GP and the complexity of the work undertaken. In the following section we examine the concept of complexity as it relates to the mental health provision within primary care. We then go on to describe a new primary care service that has been set up in City and Hackney to provide a response to the challenge of complexity by supporting GPs *and* providing a clinical service to patients. Its main aims are to bring secondary care experience into primary care; help narrow the gap in the stepped care model in a way that ensures that patients have access to the support they need, when and where they need it; and to complement existing services, particularly other primary care provision, notably as an adjunct to the local Primary Care Psychology/IAPT service.

Primary care matters

GPs and primary care surgeries are the fulcrum of the health care system in the United Kingdom. This is likely to be even more the case with the enhanced commissioning role envisaged for GPs as set out in the recent White Paper: *Equity and Excellence: Liberating the NHS* (DoH, 2010). A GP is usually the first health professional to whom people turn when they develop symptoms.[1] To illustrate the scale: the estimated average number of consultations per year *per typical practice* in London in 2008 was approximately 34,200 (Hippisley-Cox & Vinogradova, 2009).

As a generalist, one aspect of the GP's role is to link up the patient with specialist care and other resources as needed. In 2005, the Royal College of GPs called for the "development of more effective relationships and new models of care between generalist and specialist services" (RCGP, 2005, p. 7), emphasizing as essential the need to develop "long-term working relationships between generalists, specialists and lay experts" (p. 10). This fits with the stepped care model. One premise of this health care delivery framework is that patients with more complex problems, or indeed patients requiring more complex interventions (these are not necessarily synonymous), are inevitably, and perhaps always, more appropriately treated in services located higher up the stepped care system (i.e. in secondary or tertiary care). However, the reality on the ground is different. GPs do not simply function as gatekeepers, although, particularly when it comes to mental health, it is commonly thought that GPs typically manage and treat those patients with common mental health problems. This misconception should not be surprising, given the way the stepped care model functions.

Increasingly—though we would argue that this has always been more or less the case—GPs manage and treat patients with a range of complex problems, especially where there is a combination of physical and emotional factors in the presenting difficulties. The realities of primary care—and perhaps more significantly of the human condition—is that people do not necessarily fit into the referral pathways designed to manage emotional and physical difficulties. This is well conveyed by GP and systemic psychotherapist John Launer:

> The seriousness and complexity of cases seen in primary care can certainly rival that seen in any secondary or tertiary care institution. Indeed, there is an "inverse care" law at work here, which means that GPs, practice nurses, and health visitors often have to manage by themselves with the most intractable and complex cases because an onward referral is not practical or acceptable to these patients. [Launer, 2005, p. 8]

The GP and the local surgery provide a place for these patients to seek assistance. Importantly, even when patients are successfully referred on, GPs continue to hold primary responsibility and often provide ongoing support in one form or another. Patients will frequently present for help from their GPs even when they are receiving treatment elsewhere. The surgery and the GP are thus typically central pillars in the patient's and their family's life. For many the relationship with the GP provides the potential for integrated care and much-needed continuity of care over time—the qualities of care that promote physical and emotional well-being.

The unique place of the GP in the lives of patients, in turn, places particular demands on them. On the one hand, there is a curious mix of not quite knowing who will present with what problem(s) at the next consultation, encompassing a possible range of difficulties from the personal through to the social, from the physical to the emotional, allowing for the possible integration of the body and the mind. On the other hand, the GP comes to know many, if not most, patients very well, being involved at key points in their lives, often at times of crisis, working with family members and community resources over a long time span. Andrew Elder, a now retired GP who worked in primary care for over 30 years, aptly describes the importance of understanding the so-called pain of being a GP (personal communication, 2010). Professional care intersects closely with deep feelings of attachment and dependency and all the emotions, pressures, and difficulties this can arouse in both GP and patient. This dynamic shapes both the expectations with which the patients arrive and the demands that underline the GPs responses to these expectations.

Patients presenting to their GP often arrive in a state of high anxiety underlined by conscious and unconscious wishes for their needs to be fulfilled. In turn, these wishes carry the imprint of the patients' past experiences of difficult, traumatic, or neglectful earlier relationships. Patients also frequently come to see their GPs at significant times in their lives when they are facing a crisis, an illness, losses, even potentially good experiences that can be highly charged, like becoming a parent. In turn, GPs vary in their ability to manage uncertainty and contain their own and their patients' anxiety when confronted with such multilayered needs.

The emotional "costs" of this kind of work intersect with the considerable external pressures and policy shifts that erode the GP's capacity to provide this type of holistic, integrated care (Elder, 2009)—for example, the decreasing amount of time GPs have to consult with patients and the requirements to meet certain targets with attendant financial incentives or costs, say, in respect of the Quality Outcome Framework (QOF). It is likely that the planned additional responsibility for commissioning services that GPs will now be expected to assume will lead to even greater pressures on GPs in relation to patient care, though it may also be argued that the commissioning remit will provide GPs with more leverage to provide services that they believe will be more beneficial to their patients.

The nature of complexity

Taking a transdisciplinary view, Morin defines complexity as "a fabric . . . of heterogeneous constituents that are inseparably associated" (2008, p. 5). He warns that, as complexity "presents itself with the disturbing traits of a mess, of the inextricable, of disorder, of ambiguity, of uncertainty", what emerges is a need to "put phenomena in order by repressing disorder, by pushing aside the uncertain". The risk lies in the blindness to the complexity of reality that this wish to eliminate ambiguity can create. As he stresses, "[T]he difficulty of complex thought is that it must face messed . . . interconnectedness among phenomena, fogginess, uncertainty, contradiction" (2008, p. 7). What better place for a psychoanalytic approach?

In the context of mental health care, complexity can be understood on three levels: in the patients' presentation, in the interventions used to help patients with specific conditions, and in the provision of health care.

The status quo in evidence-based mental health, as reflected by the National Institute for Health and Clinical Excellence (NICE) guidelines, is dominated by a focus on patients with a single diagnosis. In this context, complexity becomes an attribute associated not with the patient, but with the intervention designed to address this isolated problem. By contrast, the reality of primary care work shows that patients present with conditions characterized by complexity, chronicity, and severity.

Patients' complexity appears as a multiplicity of mental health diagnoses, as a combination of mental and physical health problems, often coupled with a background of social difficulties, neglect, and trauma. According to Gask, Klinkman, Fortes, and Dowrick, primary care patients fall primarily into this category (2008, p. 470). Consequently, they propose to move away from relying exclusively on categorical diagnoses towards the assessment of chronicity, severity, disability, and social problems, as a source of crucial additional information that enables better targeting of interventions. Furthermore, it is important to recognize that many—if not most—of the patients seen in primary care function with sub-threshold manifestations of diagnostic categories: "like the proverbial iceberg, the greater mass of human mental pain is hidden below the diagnostic waterline" (RCGP, 2005, p. 2), a GP usually being the first health professional to whom people turn when they develop symptoms (RCGP-RCP, 2009, p. 6).

Complexity in the interventions is most commonly not reflected in the manualized therapeutic approaches on which randomized controlled trials targeted at testing efficacy are built and which then provide the evidence base for NICE guidelines. Often designed in a way that does not account for co-morbidity, research projects into the efficacy of treatments for individual diagnostic categories are at high risk of bias and carry little relevance for patients with persistent and complicated profiles. When it comes to depression and anxiety—the most common mental health complaints—very few patients experience time-limited symptoms, with both sub-threshold- and threshold-level disorders showing persistence and a tendency to evolve towards and stabilize into co-morbidity (Merikangas et al., 2003).

Furthermore, the degree of complexity encompasses complaints about both physical and mental heath. Patients with persistent medically unexplained symptoms (MUS) frequently experience depression and anxiety. Many of these patients—and often the GPs referring them—are unaware or unwilling to recognize the links between mental health on the one hand and the physical and social problems on the other.

Finally, the counterpart to complexity in terms of service provision resides in the variety of agencies with which mental health patients are engaged and the multidisciplinary nature of many of the teams that support them. The patients' complexity is also reflected in the views on and understanding of their situation as conveyed by the patients themselves, the referring GPs, and the clinicians who engage with them therapeutically.

Challenged by the difficulties that the absence of a simple explanation for or solution to their problems creates, patients often reduce the complexities of their lives to one particular condition, often of a physical nature. With this, they feel comfortable to seek help from their GPs, who, in turn, are trained to diagnose and treat clearly defined conditions. Both parties can therefore become engaged in the pursuit of a practical solution that, if found, is not likely to help. As Plsek and Greenhalgh (2001) put it when describing modern medicine: "The solution to your problem is unlikely to come in a bottle and may well involve a multidisciplinary team" (p. 625).

Such collusion is often avoided when GPs are aware of the multi-faceted problems of their patients and are able to convey this to other professionals in ways that can elicit the right kind of help. There is a degree of variability across GPs in terms of their thinking about and understanding of the mental health problems presented by patients—a point echoed by Cape and colleagues:

> [T]he more complex a GP's thinking about mental health problems is, the more likely it is that the GP will be able to help patients to make meaning of their problems in ways that may assist easing their distress and helping them engage with potentially helpful treatment. [Cape, Morris, Burd, & Buszewicz, 2008, pp. 403–404]

Responding to complexity: the City and Hackney Primary Care Psychotherapy Consultation Service

The issue of patient complexity can be addressed either by developing interventions of matching complexity or by using interventions that, by virtue of the psychotherapeutic principles on which they are based, are well placed to explore this complexity. Given its focus on the subtle—and often unconscious—underlying links between body and mind and between conceptions of the self and others, a psychoanalytically informed approach is, in our view, best placed for working with patients with multiple and varied difficulties.

It is such an approach that underpins the City and Hackney Primary Care Psychotherapy Consultation Service (PCPCS), which has developed in response to the clinical realities in primary care that we outlined earlier. Commissioned by the City and Hackney Primary Care Trust from the Tavistock and Portman NHS Foundation Trust, the service was established to support GPs with complex patients. Predominantly, three broad, sometimes overlapping, groups are catered for: people presenting with MUS, people with a diagnosis of or characteristics of a personality disorder, and people with severe and enduring mental illness. The service aims to cater for those people who do not meet the criteria for other services in primary or secondary care or who find it difficult to engage with these services. Ultimately, our patients are those who do not fit into any neat diagnostic category and whose needs cannot adequately be met within any single health or service provider.

More attention is being given to patients presenting with MUS[2] because it is an area that many GPs find perplexing and challenging, especially in light of the need for more cost-effective and better quality health care. Moreover, these patients often do not attribute their problems to their mental health and consequently do not necessarily find an understanding in these terms helpful. They are therefore less likely to be willing to access help in a mental health setting or traditional psychological therapies service. It is crucial that services and interventions are more appropriately developed to better meet the needs of these patients. However, not all patients presenting with MUS fall into the complex range, nor are all complex presentations synonymous with MUS.

There is good service provision elsewhere in the borough from the Primary Care Psychology Service (with a large IAPT component) and the secondary/tertiary care mental health Trust (psychotherapy and psychology services). While there might be some areas of overlap, the PCPCS service was established as a result of identifiable service gaps, primarily to support GPs who hold ongoing responsibility for these patients when other services seemingly have more choice in accepting or discharging patients. Although the primary basis for our involvement is the absence of another suitable service in the borough, we would see someone with the aim of supporting them to engage in services elsewhere (for example, where patients have not attended appointments offered elsewhere) or where patients are receiving a more basic level of support, say, from the local community mental health team (CMHT), and disengagement from the service would be clinically inadvisable. Often it is possible to support the GP and surgery where they are experiencing difficulties managing a patient who is engaged with another service.

Guiding principles

A large part of the work undertaken since the inception of the service has involved establishing the infrastructure, meeting GPs, and embedding our service in surgeries alongside GPs and practice staff.

Forging links and partnerships with other services from the statutory and voluntary sectors has been a priority. Our approach to developing the service has echoed our core clinical philosophy emphasizing *dialogue* and *partnership* with GPs and with patients. This places *engagement* as the essential starting point—that is, beginning with where the patient (or GP) is, rather than imposing a view or perspective on where she or he should be (Rock & Carrington, 2011).

The *multidisciplinary* team comprises professionals from psychology, psychiatry, nursing, and social work. The service is organized so that GPs have a named clinician working in their surgery to foster good local working relationships with someone familiar and accessible. Crucially, each surgery is also able to avail itself of the range of expertise and professional input from the rest of the team, as well as their named clinician, so that the provision to each surgery can be truly *multimodal* and responsive to the range of GP/patient needs. This provides for a greater span of therapeutic modes, approaches, and levels of expertise available to each surgery than simply having a stand-alone in-house professional providing psychological therapy or counselling in each surgery.

One of the distinctive features of the service has been the inclusion of principles from an *assertive outreach approach*. We do not discharge people when they do not attend appointments—something that is often the case with more high-volume services under pressure to provide greater throughput, which is often found unhelpful by GPs. We try to understand why someone might not be engaging following referral, and then we work with the GP in the service of fostering a working alliance over time. This is also helped by the fact that our clinicians work alongside GPs in surgeries and are seen as part of the "surgery umbrella". Proximity to the GP and the surgery often helps with engagement. Where appropriate, clinicians will also conduct home visits, often with the treating GP, as well as provide telephone sessions where patients are unable to travel to the surgery, usually the case when working with older patients who are physically infirm. Our DNA (Did Not Attend) rates show a reduction from 17% for first appointments to around 9% for subsequent appointments, and the service tends to engage around 94% of all patients accepted into the service at some point.

A strength of the service model, and a contribution to its added value to GPs and patients, is that interventions can be more closely matched with their specific needs rather than imposing a set of options that might not be as well suited to the presenting situation for the referrer and/or the patient. The underlying reason(s) for referring patients can be in itself complex. Patients are often referred to obtain a better understanding or formulation of a patient's difficulties or to send the patient for appropriate treatment elsewhere. The referral can also result from the GP's difficulty in managing the patient or because of the understandably intolerable feelings that can be stirred up in the GP or when a patient's situation touches on something difficult in the GP's own life, such as a bereavement.

Therefore, every referral prompts some deliberation about how we might become involved and where our involvement is best targeted: at engaging the GP, assessing the patient, working with both the GP and the patient or with the wider system, or a combination of these steps. This flexibility allows GPs in each surgery to determine to a large extent the balance and nature of our involvement depending on patient demographics, surgery lists sizes, in-house expertise, and other available services and support networks. Some GPs will draw more heavily on our resources for help with managing their patients, whereas others will refer patients for assessment and therapeutic interventions.

Our starting point when we receive a referral is a comprehensive and detailed review of the notes in order to identify relevant patterns in the patient's response to help over time. It also aids the contextualization of the current presenting problem. This information allows us to formulate the most likely beneficial care pathway and to titrate the intensity of the clinical intervention that the patient will tolerate. This is an especially relevant consideration for those people who have an experience of unhelpful previous treatments and feel that they have been passed from one service to another, which often mirrors earlier difficulties in significant attachment relationships.

Consultation to GPs

An innovative aspect of the service is that it provides a bespoke service to GPs through a combination of interventions to support the GP/surgery team. Support provided to GPs to help them manage and develop their work with their patients includes professional consultation (discussions with the GP), joint consultation (meeting with the GP and patient), case-based discussion (meeting with a group of GPs in each practice and reviewing and discussing patients), and training. We have been encouraged by the positive feedback from GPs who have engaged with these aspects of the service in feeling more able to support their patients in their surgeries. However, this remains an area for further development, as not all GPs are familiar or comfortable with this way of approaching their work.

Our service draws on a longstanding tradition in the Tavistock Clinic of working with GPs and the primary care system. The psychoanalyst Michael Balint pioneered working with GPs in groups, helping them to think about the emotional and psychological impact of the work. Balint groups, as they have come to be known, provide a reflective space in which the work of the GPs and the surgery can be shared, with a view to developing the capacity in the GPs and the surgery as a system to better treat and contain their patients. Balint's legacy has been further developed by pioneering figures such as Alexis Brook as well as, in primary care, with a focus on eye problems (Zalidis, 2009) and, in secondary care, with gastrointestinal disorders (Stern, 2009).

The aim of our joint consultation work with GPs is to assist them in thinking about their patients in ways that take complexity into account, thus enabling them to relate to their patients so as to facilitate their future engagement and communication. In the words of Cape and colleagues:

> In many cases, "simpler" rather than complex explanations may be more useful to patients. However, it can be hypothesised that the more complex the GP's psychosocial thinking about the patient, the more likely it is that the GP will be able to come up with an explanation that fits, is acceptable to the patient, and helps them to feel less distressed, and more understood, and more able to deal with their problems. [Cape et al., 2008, p. 408]

Given the centrality of the GP–patient relationship, these interventions are often focused on effecting some change that can lead to a shift in the dynamics between the GP and the patient, thus leading to some development. This might mean the GP being better able to identify a way forward that had not been apparent before, such as a referral to another service or involving another professional from the surgery team, or it might result in the GP having greater confidence in holding the patient in the surgery and recognizing the limits of what is possible. We are also interested in helping patients to manage their difficulties in ways that will, hopefully, influence their help-seeking behaviour and their relationships elsewhere, leading to more productive outcomes.

In a recent survey of GPs using our service, most respondents reported feeling more able to refer appropriately to other services as well as to feeling more able to manage these patients themselves without onward referral. This is consistent with GPs being more able to manage the feelings expressed by their patients and to gain a more detailed understanding of the emotional dynamics driving the behaviour of their patients and the unfolding relationship with their GP and others.

Joint consultations can be effective in enabling GPs to recover their capacity to remain involved and sympathetic to the patient's predicament, especially when they feel tested or pushed to their emotional and/or professional limits. These feelings and capacities can be severely challenged when seemingly intractable or at least repetitive difficulties arise with specific patients in consultations, bringing with them a familiar sinking feeling in the GP.

"Heartsink consultations"

The term "heartsink patient" is an established part of the lexicon of general practice. Growing out of the experiences described by O'Dowd (1988), it conveys the so-called sinking of the heart feeling in the face of helplessness, frustration, and difficulty experienced by the health professional. GPs can also feel unprofessional (Butler et al., 1999); this, in our experience, is sometimes related to feeling unable to help patients in the way that is expected.

It is interesting to note that in some of the original work instigated by O'Dowd (as described in an excellent discussion paper by Butler et al., 1999) to support GPs to better manage their "heartsink" experiences—arranging meetings to discuss the patients, share information, and support the treating clinician—those patients who were discussed consulted their GPs less frequently. In this group, these patients tended to see the same GP, compared with the group who had not been discussed.[3] O'Dowd's work provides evidence that a forum where GPs can discuss their experiences and be supported improves their feelings and the care provided, thereby making it more possible to manage better both their feelings and those of the patient. The PCPCS was developed to support these forums and to use joint consultations with individual GPs to provide an additional perspective that might shift some of the more enduring complications.

Butler et al. (1999) point out the seriousness of the phenomenon in general practice and cite various figures from other studies to show its prevalence. Given the pejorative connotations of the term "heartsink patient" because it implies that all the difficulties come from the patient, we prefer the term "heartsink consultations"[4] because it gives emphasis to the fact that often both GPs and patients alike share feelings of frustration and dissatisfaction at not being able to help or be helped. "Heartsink consultations" result from a number of factors, including patient- and clinician-influenced variables, though it is frequently the result of an interaction between the patient and clinician.

From a psychoanalytic perspective, it is possible to understand some of the prevailing dynamics in terms of the nature of any therapeutic encounter that inevitably has an emotional or psychological impact on the professional too, without him or her necessarily being aware of the impact. Freud wrote, "It is a very remarkable thing that the unconscious of one human being can react upon that of another, without passing through the conscious" (1915e, p. 194).

Possible difficulties arise when these dynamics go unrecognized and therefore unaddressed. Given that the PCPCS deals with the more complex end of the clinical spectrum, it is not surprising that we often become involved at a point at which something has become stuck between the patient and the GP and/or other professionals in the system.

Clinical service

The PCPCS also provides a direct clinical service. In our experience the combination of a clinical service with the mediated approach offered to GPs is particularly beneficial to GPs and patients. It also allows for augmented provision at different times, in keeping with another principle of the stepped care model: providing the minimum intervention to effect change. Further interventions can be offered without having to refer the patient to another service for a new treatment episode with all the possible difficulties of engagement and reassessment.

One hallmark of the PCPCS is the provision of comprehensive assessments to guide treatment choice. Individual, couple, and group therapy are provided, with various models being drawn on, such as dynamic interpersonal therapy (DIT), CBT, supportive psychotherapy, and mentalization-based treatment (MBT). Because part of the service remit is to see patients with MUS, we have developed specific psycho-educational groups for people who speak English and for people who speak Turkish.[5]

Case management is another intervention in the service to facilitate better engagement with appropriate statutory/voluntary services or community resources. The service also provides help with *signposting* to other more suitable services. Most of our interventions are delivered in a brief, structured manner for up to 16 sessions. However, this can be offered across a range of frequencies, depending on the needs of the patient and referrer.

Regardless of the nature of the intervention, it is the same psychoanalytic ethos that underpins the clinical thinking—an ability to make and keep connections in mind and a tolerance of uncertainty. This arises in relation to the complexity that patients bring and the desire of both patient and GP to pin it down to a specific treatable condition—and sometimes the inability to do so. Not knowing what is wrong can create great anxieties in the patient. Not being able to find an immediate and concrete answer can trigger equally great anxieties in the GP. Our role is not to provide a new diagnostic category in which GPs can fit their patients, but to help them both to recognize and tolerate this uncertainty and the impact it has on their relationship. Furthermore, a psychoanalytic approach helps by providing an understanding of the dynamics in significant relationships linked to attachment styles and early formative influences as well as an understanding of how anxieties and wishes are stimulated in emotionally significant relationships (with the threats and opportunities that this poses). This includes an understanding of the contribution of transference phenomena, countertransference, and the inevitable pull to the re-enactment of previously unsatisfying, frustrating, or hurtful relationship experiences.

The following two brief clinical vignettes demonstrate the PCPCS' approach to two different clinical presentations.[6]

Clinical vignette 1

This clinical vignette gives an example of the utility of having some options in meeting the patient at the point of coming for psychological help. It illustrates the value of conducting a more thorough psychological assessment that proved helpful in later re-establishing a better contact between the GP and the patient, thereby supporting a needed system of care following a suicide attempt:

> Joanne had long-standing difficulties with depression and presented to her GP every three or four months. She was in her mid-thirties and had two young children to look after. She often felt overwhelmed and unable to cope with their felt demands. She was also concerned about her teenage son from a previous relationship. He had begun to behave in "strange" ways that made her worry about his ability to see out his last year at school. He was becoming very withdrawn and secretive.

> Joanne had been referred for counselling before and had not found it helpful. So, when the GP referred her to the local IAPT service, she simply did not attend appointments and was discharged. After referral to our service, we suggested having a joint meeting with the GP, whom Joanne had known for a fairly long time, and the patient. At this meeting she agreed to meet with the clinician on her own. On her own, she talked about thoughts of harming herself when she felt especially frustrated. She also harboured thoughts of killing herself and felt that her children would be better off without her. When she felt so low and despairing, she also felt more aggrieved because at these times she felt that no one had really been there for her. In the course of the work, the clinician helped Joanne's son to get help of his own through the local services. It was at this point that Joanne said that she did not feel that she needed any more regular appointments for herself. The clinician kept contacting Joanne to keep contact with her and kept in regular contact with the GP.

> In the course of events, Joanne made a serious suicide attempt. She did not contact her GP or the clinician beforehand or follow the risk plan that had been put in place for her. The GP then discovered that Joanne had reported to A&E that her GP was very unsupportive. He was rather surprised and upset by this and

began questioning whether he should continue to offer her help in the surgery.

The clinician was in a position to describe the patient's state of mind with a better sense of her feelings of grievance that originated in her relationship with her own parents, who had been felt to abandon her when she was a teenager. In turn, the GP was able to better understand the extent to which Joanne's perception of him, which was usually positive, had become distorted by her distress and sense of crisis. This enabled him to become more engaged with her and put their professional relationship on a better footing, especially helping him to appreciate the seriousness of her depressive episodes.

The clinician was able to engage the patient by partnering with the treating GP and then by gaining a more in-depth formulation of the patient's sense of abandonment and grievance during a time of crisis—importantly, when the patient was helped to get support for her son, about whom she was worried. The extent to which her concerns for him also conveyed and masked her own emotional disturbance was a factor that was used to help the GP better understand the reasons why she might have acted in the way she did. Keeping some contact with the patient, in spite of Joanne's decision not to attend individual appointments, enabled a greater responsiveness from our service and the GP when things took a turn for the worse. Although this sadly did not prevent her from attempting to take her life, it was possible to assist the GP through a more developed formulation to go on engaging with the patient.

Clinical vignette 2

This vignette shows a breakdown in the patient's functioning following a consultation with a medical specialist, who was giving the patient a "realistic" view of the prognosis, which might be understood as a reaction to a "heartsink consultation" and the PCPCS' subsequent involvement.

Mark was referred for long-standing non-epileptic attack disorder. Now, in his late thirties, Mark felt considerable despair of ever getting better. This feeling had been exacerbated by a recent medical examination in which he had been advised to expect a worsening of his condition over time. Mark's condition was already profoundly debilitating: he rarely left his flat, was socially isolated apart from a cousin who had taken on the role of carer, and was unable to carry out basic daily living functions. As a result of feeling so pessimistic about his future, Mark made plans to take his own life. He was referred by his GP when his carer discovered that he had been hoarding prescription sleeping tablets with a view to taking an overdose and "ending it all".

Our involvement started with an extensive review of his medical and psychiatric notes. It was noted that Mark had had extensive input from a range of mental health professionals: he had received CBT for anxiety, group therapy (including therapy for his specific condition), and individual counselling. He had been seen by the local CMHT. None of this had been felt to be very helpful.

The work with Mark began with the impact of his experience of his debilitating symptoms, as he was having daily "attacks". Mark was confused about his various diagnoses and thought that perhaps he had always experienced epilepsy and had now developed non-epileptic attacks that continued to coexist. There was no medical evidence for this, as, on investigation, no abnormal EEG activity had been found.

Initially Mark was extremely reluctant to talk about his life, relationships, or any other significant experiences. The clinician working with him began to use his own feelings of being shut out by him to begin to articulate Mark's possible need to keep others and the world at bay for fear of experiences becoming too intrusive from his point of view and therefore emotionally overwhelming. Although this functioned to protect Mark, it was also stopping him from engaging in more fruitful relationships with others that he also wanted to have. Tentatively, a link was also made with Mark's presenting symptoms and the extent to which his fits—in which he often lost consciousness—both concealed and showed the extent of his feelings, especially his anger.

Of course, for someone like Mark, who has experienced significant difficulties over a long period, there was no dramatic change, but over the course of the work his symptoms decreased significantly.

He also reported feeling less suicidal and, importantly, began to take steps to reconnect with some friends to lessen his social isolation.

Evaluating complexity

Under the influence of the Medical Research Council's definition of the "gold standard" of evidence, the prevailing approach to psychotherapy research is to focus on the treatment of patients with specific diagnostic conditions—such as depression. While randomized controlled trials (RCTs) involving homogenous patients are presented as the framework to aspire to, it is recognized that the patients included in such studies are not representative of the majority of patients referred for psychotherapy and even less so of patients seen daily in GP surgeries, with their multiple symptoms and chronic complaints. Guthrie argues that "studies of psychotherapy should have clinical relevance, and should be targeted towards definable clinical populations or characteristics of patients, rather than diagnostic conditions" (2000, p. 131). This is consistent with patient-centred as opposed to illness-centred approach, a paradigm shift that may be well supported by the limitations of the current mainstream approaches in the context of mental health.

Sir Michael Rawlins, Chairman of NICE since its inception, is, however, among the most prominent voices to warn against mechanistic approaches to the assessment of evidence, where the single aim of the exercise is to inform decision makers about the appropriate use of therapeutic interventions in routine clinical practice. While recognizing the merits of RCTs, he stresses that "[H]ierarchies of evidence should be replaced by accepting—indeed embracing—a diversity of approaches" (Rawlins, 2008, p. 34).

One criticism often levelled at the efficacy shown in RCTs is that the conditions under which the interventions take place are not representative, with the therapists delivering them being usually highly skilled and experienced—more so than in everyday clinical practice. Consistently, the preliminary results after the first year of the IAPT initiative indicate that better patient outcomes correlate significantly with higher level of therapist experience (Glover, Webb, & Evison, 2010, p. 38). On these grounds, we can hypothesize that by design the

PCPCS is well placed to facilitate noticeable outcome changes. At the same time, it is likely that these improvements would be mitigated by the short nature of the interventions, with a J-curve effect to be expected as patients' awareness of their own difficulties heightens their distress before it enables them to work through the problems they face. An added challenge to a meaningful evaluation relates to the multidimensional nature of change and the notorious difficulties inherent in multidimensional comparisons.

Drawing on the theory of complex systems, Plsek and Greenhalgh stress the importance of interdependence in health care: "Since each agent and each system is nested within other systems, all evolving together and interacting, we cannot fully understand any of the agents or systems without reference to the others" (2001, p. 626).

An important implication of this understanding of the reality of mental health is that evaluation becomes very difficult. Given that "no part of the equation is constant, independent, or predictable" (Plsek & Greenhalgh, 2001, p. 625), "the only way to know exactly what a complex system will do is to observe it: it is not a question of better understanding the agents, of better models, or of more analysis" (p. 627). This therefore requires a broader conceptualization of the outcomes sought and the ways of gathering realistic and meaningful data.

Such constraints on evaluation pose great difficulties in relation to the expectation of accountability that comes with providing mental health services that are publicly funded. While recognizing the pitfalls of oversimplification and of a reductionist stance, it is essential that we remain able to gauge the value of the service we provide to all concerned—patients, GPs, and commissioners alike. Consequently we have developed a data-monitoring strategy that incorporates four main domains: process evaluation, client satisfaction, outcome evaluation, and economic evaluation. All combine quantitative and qualitative methods.

The process evaluation is concerned with monitoring and assessing the processes involved in setting up the service and anchoring it to the reality of primary care. This is an ongoing project. The client satisfaction component aims to capture the experience of both GPs and patients accessing the service. Responses are currently being collected in an online questionnaire for City and Hackney GPs (briefly mentioned in the previous section), while a patient satisfaction questionnaire is being finalized. Outcome evaluation is devoted to assessing changes through measures that capture patients' mental health and general functioning. Data is also being collected on measures of distress and quality of life for a subset of patients, in view of a forthcoming quantitative analysis.

Finally, the economic evaluation component concentrates on estimating associated direct and indirect costs and benefits. Its main focus is on changes in the envisaged reduction in pressure on GP surgery resources from frequent attenders. Particularly, the high volume of medical investigations, admissions, and interventions is assessed by reviewing the changes in the number of GP, secondary care, and A&E appointments these patients make in the 12 months prior to engagement with PCPCS and the 12 months following discharge from our service. This is most salient in the current financial climate, where the imperative is to provide better quality services for less money.

Conclusion

Our starting point was the recognition that primary care is central to a health care system that engages with patients presenting with complex clinical and socioeconomic profiles. The level of complexity confronted daily in GP surgeries requires that a flexible approach is taken, one that places the patient at its core and builds on the crucial role of the patient–GP relationship.

Conceived with these key ideas in mind, the PCPCS works as an integral part of the primary care system in City and Hackney, offering a flexible and multimodal approach, anchored by a broadly psychoanalytic perspective. We provide a variety of intervention options that cover both assessment and treatment, ensuring that experienced clinicians are available from the outset of the referral pathway.

An innovation of the service is the direct input to GPs, enabling them to support their more complex patients both to recognize and to navigate through inevitable emotional difficulties. GPs and patients alike value this approach, as illustrated in both the direct feedback received and the improved engagement reflected in our DNA rates.

This is an illustration of how the issue of patient complexity can be addressed using interventions that, by virtue of the psychotherapeutic principles on which they are based, are well placed to explore this complexity. Some of these principles are intrinsically linked to the psychotherapeutic tradition developed by the Tavistock Clinic. If the PCPCS is to offer a relevant service model adequate to the task of supporting complex clinical realities in primary care, it must continue to draw on this tradition. At the same time, the experience of delivering the service shows us that engaging with this reality requires not only strong theoretical and clinical foundations, but also a flexible approach and an ability to balance continuity with change, in a way that takes the inherent pressures and opportunities into account.

Notes

1. Their importance is acknowledged in the joint report by the Royal College of General Practitioners and the Royal College of Psychiatrists (RCGP-RCP, 2009).

2. According to Webb, MUS "refers to symptoms and signs of physical distress or malfunction that cannot be accounted for by any physical disorder a patient is known to have. It includes both symptoms in the absence of apparent illness, and the emergence of severe symptoms in those who have only mild illness. . . . [It excludes] those symptoms caused by physical illness that has yet to be discovered, though inevitably there will be an unknowable but small proportion in this category" (Webb, 2010, p. 4).

3. This is very similar to some of the guidance emerging from the Commissioning Support for London MUS pilot project. One aspect is for specific GPs to take responsibility for specific patients and offer these patients regular appointments at specified intervals to better coordinate and integrate care (CSL, 2010).

4. A term coined by Matthew Patrick, Chief Executive of the Tavistock and Portman NHS Foundation Trust.

5. This is offered in partnership with the local Turkish counselling organization, Derman (www.derman.org.uk).

6. All identifying details have been changed for the purpose of confidentiality.

References

Butler, C. C., Evans, M., & the Welsh Philosophy and General Practice Discussion Group (1999). The "heartsink" patient revisited. *British Journal of General Practice, 49* (440): 230–233.

Cape, J., Morris, E., Burd, M., & Buszewicz, M. (2008). Complexity of GPs' explanations about mental health problems: Development, reliability and validity of a measure. *British Journal of General Practice, 58*: 403–410.

CSL (2010). *Medically Unexplained Symptoms (MUS): A Whole Systems Approach*. London: Commissioning Support for London. Available at: www.londonhp.nhs.uk/wp-content/uploads/2011/03/MUS-whole-systems-approach.pdf

DoH (2010). *Equity and Excellence: Liberating the NHS*. London: Department of Health/The Stationery Office. Available at: www.dh.gov.uk/health/search/?searchTerms=Liberating+the+NHS

Elder, A. (2009). Building on the work of Alexis Brook: Further thoughts about brief psychotherapy in primary care. *Psychoanalytic Psychotherapy, 23* (4): 307–320.

Freud, S. (1915e). The unconscious. *Standard Edition*, 14: 166–215.

Gask, L., Klinkman, M., Fortes, S., & Dowrick, C. (2008). Capturing complexity: The case for a new classification system for mental disorders in primary care. *European Psychiatry, 23*: 469–476.

Glover, G., Webb, M., & Evison, F. (2010). *Improving Access to Psychological Therapies: A Review of the Progress Made by Sites in the First Rollout Year*. Stockton on Tees: North East Public Health Observatory. Available at: www.wmrdc.org.uk/silo/files/iapt-year-1-sites-data-review-final-report.pdf

Guthrie, E. (2000). Psychotherapy for patients with complex disorders and chronic symptoms. *British Journal of Psychiatry, 177*: 131–137.

Hippisley-Cox, J., & Vinogradova, Y. (2009). *Trends in Consultation Rates in General Practice 1995 to 2008: Analysis of the QResearch® Database. Final Report to the NHS Information Centre and Department of Health*. London: Department of Health.

Launer, J. (2005). Introduction. In: J. Launer, S. Blake, & D. Daws (Eds.), *Reflecting on Reality: Psychotherapists at Work in Primary Care* (pp. 1–17). London: Karnac.

Merikangas, R. K., Zhang, H., Avenevoli, S., Acharyya, S., Neuenschwander, M., & Angst, J. (2003). Longitudinal trajectories of depression and anxiety in a prospective community study. *Archives of General Psychiatry, 60*: 993–1000.

Morin, E. (2008). *On Complexity*. Cresskill, NJ: Hampton Press.

O'Dowd, T. C. (1988). Five years of heartsink patients in general practice. *British Medical Journal, 297*: 528–530.

Plsek, P. E., & Greenhalgh, T. (2001). The challenge of complexity in health care. *British Medical Journal, 323*: 625–628.

Rawlins, M. (2008). *De Testimonio: On the Evidence for Decisions about the Use of Therapeutic Interventions*. The Harveian Oration. London: Royal College of Physicians.

RCGP (2005). *Royal College of General Practitioners Position Statement: Mental Health and Primary Care*. Arising from the RCGP Health Inequalities Standing Group Conference held jointly with the National Institute for Mental Health in England (NIMHE), entitled Hard Lives: Living with Mental Health Inequalities, Birmingham, 26 March 2004. London: Royal College of General Practitioners.

RCGP-RCP (2009). *The Management of Patients with Physical and Psychological Problems in Primary Care: A Practical Guide*. Report of a joint working group of the Royal College of General Practitioners and the Royal College of Psychiatrists. London: Royal College of Psychiatrists.

Rock, B., & Carrington, A. (2011). Addressing complexity in primary care. *Healthcare Counselling & Psychotherapy Journal*, 11 (1): 35–39.

Stern, J. (2009). Keeping the gut in mind. *Psychoanalytic Psychotherapy*, 23 (4): 330–339.

Webb, T. (2010). Why we need to address medically unexplained symptoms. *Healthcare Counselling & Psychotherapy Journal*, 10 (1): 4–8.

Zalidis, S. (2009). Tears: Emotional or somatic? *Psychoanalytic Psychotherapy*, 23 (4): 321–329.

CHAPTER SIX

Treatment continuity in discontinuous worlds

Carine Minne

Long-term continuity of treatment for forensic patients: a luxury or necessity?

In this chapter, I present the case of a very ill young man who, in addition to the usual psychiatric treatment, was provided with long-term continuity of psychoanalytic psychotherapy during the ten years he spent moving from a high secure psychiatric setting and eventually back to the community. The provision of such long-term psychotherapy for patients suffering from serious mental disorders can be misconstrued as a luxury. The NICE Guideline (2009) that maps out treatment for patients in forensic psychiatry settings has, for example, recognized the need to lengthen interventions, but these can remain disrupted as the patient moves between clinical teams and may, accordingly, be concerned with short-term goals of "treating crises, symptoms of distress . . . rather than core personality disorder psychopathology" (Warren, 2003). Furthermore, the economic consid-erations on public health-care spending have focused the attention away from what the patient fully requires to what is cost-effective. Published research has substantiated the need to reconsider the treat-ments typically given to severely disturbed patients; a meta-analysis of studies of the phenomenon of psychopathy found longer-lasting treatments more effective, albeit this included anything over as little as one year long (Salekin, 2002). The paper also indicates that recidivism in cases where continuous care is absent costs significantly to the community.

In my view, the provision of long-term therapy for these patients is not a luxury but, rather, a necessity, paramount to recovery, and, furthermore, is likely to be more cost-effective than short-term limited treatments. It may be helpful to make an analogy with diabetes, a chronic and debilitating physical illness, which can be controlled with continuous long-term treatment and monitoring. The kinds of mental disorders I will refer to are also chronic and debilitating and could be considered as "diabetes of the mind" in terms of their endurance and the extent to which they debilitate. The case study will be used to highlight the value of appropriate therapeutic frameworks within long-term continuous care and also to explain how a particular diagnostic tool (the Operationalised Psychodynamic Diagnostics—OPD) can offer the psychotherapist, as well as the wider clinical team, an understanding of patients, their requirements, and the impact of interpersonal relating. Furthermore, this tool can be used to monitor treatment progress and assess what, if any, mental structural changes have arisen, and these will also be described.

Patients treated in forensic psychiatry settings are invariably people who suffer from severe mental disorders and have seriously offended. They are expected to recover, move through the system (down the levels of security), and end up living back in the community. There are many other psychiatric patients who do not end up treated in forensic psychiatry settings but are also severely ill and expected to eventually manage living in the community. Many of these patients eventually come under the care of overstretched community mental health teams (CMHTs) or even one of the rare forensic CMHTs. The patients seen in forensic psychiatry settings often come from dysfunctional families, and many have spent time in a variety of care settings or penal and/or other psychiatric institutions. They have often had harsh and cruel experiences in their early years, which have affected the development of their personalities and their interpersonal relations. Their attachment capacities, and hence their ability to form therapeutic relationships, are usually severely damaged and maladaptive.

What is particularly striking is the degree to which these patients have never received adequate care by a consistent figure, either in early childhood or later, at home or within an institution. With our current system of care, the care may be adequate but there is a risk of repetition of these earlier experiences of numerous changes in parental figures. Often these patients' first experience of consistent adequate care comes as a result of a catastrophe—their index offence—leading to a relatively lengthy admission in a forensic psychiatric secure setting. This can be the ideal time to engage such people in psychotherapy, one aim being to enable them to develop the capacity to form trusting relationships for the first time by offering them a forum to work psychoanalytically within a therapeutic relationship.

Under the present system, forensic psychiatry services are structured in such a way that when a patient starts to improve and is considered ready to move to conditions of lesser security, that patient's geographical placement usually changes entirely. So too does their clinical team. In other words, once these patients have benefited from consistent, adequate care over a period of months or years, a complete change in care transpires. This can inflame earlier experiences of loss, abandonment, and betrayal, with consequent distress. Such distress can cause deterioration in the patient's mental state and even a regression to previous functioning. This can mean a raised risk of the need to "act out": to rid oneself of unwanted or unbearable feelings. Alternatively, the patient quietly suffers from a depressed state of mind, having to face the anxious transition period of losing everything he or she has become familiar with and managing the sense of grief that can arise. Those states of mind can be camouflaged through a sense of shame experienced at feeling the loss or alternatively by achieving states of manic denial.

It was with this in mind that I allocated a small number of patients in a high-security hospital for psychoanalytic psychotherapy, which would continue to be provided by the same therapist, myself, across the different levels of security until and including when they were back in the community. These patients also continued to receive the usual therapeutic treatment plans, including CBT and group therapy. The thinking behind long-term continuous therapy was twofold. First, at each move towards the community, anxiety levels are raised with the risk of regressed states of mind; consequently, there is an increased risk of enactment either towards the self or towards another. Providing ongoing psychotherapy within an ever-stronger therapeutic relationship would maximize the chance of a smoother transition from one placement to the other. In other words, a safe thinking space would be maintained to address any difficult feelings engendered. Second, the mental disorders many of these patients suffer from are known to be chronic and deeply engrained and mainly within the personality disorders category. This, in my view, necessitates the long-term provision of at least the psychoanalytic psychotherapy component of the overall treatment, as it enables the personality difficulties to be seriously addressed and to allow real internal world changes to take place—not simply a noted behavioural improvement with a stable mental state within the context of the secure and containing setting provided. Furthermore, I would argue that, as the level of physical security diminishes, the level of therapeutic input should in some cases be increased. This can help patients to gradually shift from remaining "well" within a containing external physical environment to relying on a containing "internal" one.

The proposals described above were designed in keeping with a number of recommendations in policies that emerged over the last two decades regarding the treatments of people suffering from personality disorders. The Reed Report (Reed, 1992), the Ashworth Enquiry (Fallon, Blugrass, Edwards, & Daniels, 1999), and the Tilt Report (Tilt, Perry, Martin, Maguire, & Preston, 2000) all recommended that psychodynamic psychotherapy be made available to these patients within secure psychiatric institutions. These proposals were also in keeping with the National Service Framework Guidelines regarding patients with severe disorders having access to appropriate treatments (DoH, 2009; NICE, 2009). These proposals are in keeping with what has been learnt in one hundred years of psychoanalytic work regarding: the development of the mind and the impact of adverse circumstances, the treatment of personality disorders, attachment theory, and the importance of working transferentially for internal changes to take root firmly.

Case illustration

I will illustrate the long-term psychotherapy treatment of a forensic psychiatry patient across different levels of security, from high, medium, to low, until he was ready to return to live in the community.

At the age of 17 years, Mr C killed his mother and was convicted of manslaughter. He was detained in hospital for nine years under a Hospital Order from the court. He was in high security for the first seven years, in medium security for the following two years, and was discharged to the community the following year.

Mr C grew up in a very deprived part of London. He is the eldest of three sons by his teenage mother's relationship that broke down when they were very young, which resulted in no further contact with the father. Mr C's mother was seriously alcoholic and described in one social worker's report as "preferring a can of beer to her own children". She neglected her children, herself, and her home. There are descriptions of her repeatedly telling her children they were "a piece of shit". For Mr C to be told this may have led to the belief that his mother could only produce shit, and this has had strong implications in the transference, especially early on, when I, his psychotherapist, was suspected by the patient of dressing up as a therapist/mother when all I would offer him was "shit".

Mr C truanted frequently, but it was not until he was 9 years old that he was referred to professionals because of behavioural problems. He then attended a special school for disturbed boys, but this school also expelled him. Between 10 and 12 years of age he ran away from home regularly, lived on the streets, and belonged to a gang of older boys who took drugs and committed burglaries. This was a boy with a totally dysfunctional existence, with no parental guidance whatsoever.

When he was 12 years old, his mother was asked to bring him to a Family Court. He apparently felt anxious that he was going to be taken away into care and asked his mother for reassurance. She told him not to worry, she would not let them do this, and that she would look after him. When it was his mother's turn to speak in court, she began complaining bitterly about how awful he was and how she could not cope with him, and she asked the court to take him away. This is in fact the moment, I think, when his mother received, unbeknown to either of them, her death sentence.

Mr C was placed in different care homes, all of which he kept running away from. Due to ongoing absconding, he was sent to a long-term children's home far from London, where he stayed for three years. This was the most settled period to date in his life, and there he thrived, socially and academically. After turning 16, he was promoted to a "cluster flat" within this children's home, to acknowledge increasing capacity for independence. He was thrilled by this but experienced it as a stressful demand. He dealt with his inability to manage this by burgling another one of the cluster flats. He was charged and taken to court, where the outcome of the case was, astonishingly, that he was forbidden to return to the home; instead, the probation officer was to give him a train ticket back to London. He was told in court that he did not deserve what had been offered to him. Therefore, he left the children's home with no preparation whatsoever. As he fell in a service provision gap for 16- to 18-year-olds, he had no choice but to return to stay at his mother's flat. Within two months, she was dead.

On the day of the killing, he had been drinking heavily with his mother since early morning. They ran out of alcohol after several hours, and she insisted that he go out to buy some more. A row ensued, during which she repeatedly called him a piece of shit. At this moment, against the background of experiencing the rejection by the children's home, his illusion of shared time with a drinking mate/mother may have shattered when he realized he was only her means of getting alcohol—in other words, merely an object to satisfy her. He told me that he could not tolerate the demands she was making, and he "cracked up" and attacked her. She fell unconscious to the floor, and he believed that she was feigning being dead. He proceeded to attack her ferociously in his psychotic state of belief that she was still a danger to his survival, until she was obliterated. He then slept in the same room, woke up the next morning, stepped over her body, and went out to the shops, even buying alcohol for her. Later that day he was arrested. He denied having killed his mother, and it is likely that he believed this, as he appears to have been in a dissociated state, which enabled him to go to sleep and to get up the next morning as though nothing had happened.

On admission to a high-security hospital, Mr C was noted to be impulsive, abusive, jovial, or clowning around and always pushing boundaries. He started to attend some treatment programmes and work centres, but this was considered to be compliant behaviour on his part with one objective: to get out. This detachment from any truth about himself and his history was maintained until he started psychoanalytic psychotherapy, which was his first experience of being with a person who showed consistent interest in him and repeatedly questioned his laughing and joking things off, considering how serious the predicament was for a young man, himself, in this hospital for having killed his mother. Slowly, Mr C began to take himself more seriously. He gradually discovered that he had a thing called a mind that he could make use of.

Early on, sessions with me began with a chirpy jocular entrance and an attempt to turn my visit into a social one, and far away from anything serious. If I interpreted his use of jokiness as a defence against seriousness, he could experience this as too demanding. When demands became too much, he had to get rid of these, stop me affecting him, just like he stopped his mother. He would ask me to shut up and, eventually, was able to describe the violent fantasies about me that filled his mind at those moments.

Another feature that came up was his tendency to become high, even without actual drugs available. He would, for example, deprive himself of sleep the night before his sessions in order to feel high during them. He could not yet trust himself to be sad and needed his manic defence desperately, increasingly so as I interpreted this to him.

His developing sense of curiosity in himself and diminution in his terror of his "mad" parts were impressive. He gradually became able to experience me as a good object but not perfect—in other words, not idealized in his previously manic world but not a demonized shit-producer either. In a session just before he left high security, he came calmly into the room, sat down, and told me that he had moved rooms and had spent all the previous day cleaning out his new room thoroughly. It had been absolutely filthy to start off with and was now much cleaner, but there was still a bit to go. I nodded with an expression indicating "yes, we know about that". His grin indicated that he understood. He then told me that there had been an incident, which had troubled him. A patient who wanted a chat had come to his door while he was cleaning the new room and sat down outside it. The patient had lit a cigarette, and Mr C noticed this, knowing it to be against the rules, but he said nothing, although he felt uncomfortable as it was right outside his door. Two nurses checking the corridor area noticed the smoking and immediately came to tell the other patient that this was forbidden and took him away. One of those nurses came back to Mr C and accused him of having offered the light. He felt furious by this accusation and said that he would have in the past, but not any more. His protests of innocence were ignored. They did not believe him. He then looked up at me questioningly. I said that he was very upset that the nurses, and maybe I too, still thought of him as how he used to be and not how he feels himself to be now: much "cleaner", but still a way to go.

Continuity in therapy and therapist, given Mr C's particular history of inconsistencies, abandonments, and losses, was particularly important. This was a young man who had never been able to experience sad feelings but had, instead, developed a formidable manic repertoire to defend against these, which had failed him miserably and tragically. Continuity offered him the opportunity to further develop his internal world shifts towards a healthier way of responding to external events, particularly those reminiscent of earlier experiences. The move from high security, agreed by professionals after seven years, albeit highly desired by him, like the promotion to the cluster flat earlier, was complicated by the additional experience of feeling abandoned or even betrayed by high security, as he had been by the residential home and, earlier still, by his mother. The difference was that he was able to recognize his states of mind and speak about the feelings engendered this time. Just before leaving high security, he said to me: "You know, I'm so pleased to have made it to this stage and be moving on, but there is a part of me that would like to simply live in a nice little cottage in the grounds of this high-security hospital. Then I could be sure you and the team had not overestimated me, and if things went wrong, I'd still be in the right place." Simultaneously, the patient had to manage experiencing guilt due to his capacity for remorse and for having got better, which led him to periodically feel suicidal.

After one year of me travelling weekly to see him in his new medium-secure unit, he obtained Home Office permission to come escorted to the Portman Clinic for sessions. On his first occasion of coming to see me, he said, upon entering my consulting room, "Wow, it's great to come and see you, to be here, at last—we MADE it!"—a not untypical manic response to feeling anxious. Eventually, after several months, he had Home Office permission to make the journey alone. This "promotion" led to the first of several minor re-enactments. After this particular session, instead of travelling straight back to the medium-secure unit, he deviated to his old home territory and met up with past "colleagues" who celebrated his visit with alcohol and the offer of "work". He then telephoned me in an intoxicated state, asking for help. The situation was dealt with immediately, and he was safely back in the medium-secure unit a few hours later. I interpreted what had happened to him in his next session not just as his re-enactment of how he responded to earlier "promotions", but also as his way of checking to see if he had indeed changed and also seeking reassurance that his old self was alive and kicking. This one incident took several months of sessions to be dissected and understood.

This patient was subsequently discharged to his own flat, attended evening college, worked during the day, and travelled a long distance every week for his psychotherapy sessions.

The Operationalised Psychodynamic Diagnostics formulation system

Probably the most important aspect the long-term continuity of treatment provided this patient was a constant reliable object who remained available throughout this enforced treatment period, which arose only because of the catastrophe that had occurred. I will try to illustrate how the developments in his mental states, and also in his mental structure, arose; I describe these using the OPD Formulation system (OPD Task Force, 2001).

The OPD system was developed by a group of psychiatrists, psychoanalysts, and psychotherapists in Germany in the early 1990s as a result of the state at that time of psychoanalytic diagnostics and a general dissatisfaction with the phenomenological approaches of classification available in DSM–III (APA, 1980) and the ICD–10 (WHO, 1992). The system was developed as a way of capturing the essence of psychodynamic constructs close to observation, thereby complementing phenomenological diagnostics. It was set up along five main axes. Axes II, III, and IV were derived from the concepts of transference and countertransference, intrapsychic conflict, and personality structure; Axis V is a phenomenological classification, linking directly with DSM and ICD. The axes are named as follows:

I   experience of illness and prerequisites for treatment;
II   interpersonal relations;
III   conflict;
IV   mental structure;
V   mental and psychosomatic disorders.

The system was developed with the intention

1.   to provide clinical diagnostic guidelines that, by virtue of their relatively open formulation, allows users enough scope for their own assessments;
2.   to be useful for training in psychodynamic psychotherapy, providing practice in both psychodynamic and phenomenological classification;
3.   to improve communication within the scientific community regarding psychodynamic constructs;
4.   to be used for scientific research.

I will illustrate the progressive changes at salient moments in Mr C's long-term treatment, emphasizing this with reference mainly to Axes I, II, and IV of the OPD system.

Upon his admission to the high-security hospital, an experience of being ill was almost absent in Mr C, and he presented himself, not unusually for an adolescent in a forensic psychiatric setting of this kind, as being there with one thing in mind: to get out as fast as possible. He appeared not to be in touch at all with the fact of being a psychiatric patient with a serious mental disorder who needed treatment in a high-security hospital, nor of being aware of the fact that he had killed his mother. Rather, Mr C presented himself as an adolescent boy clowning around and trying to turn every encounter into a joke. For example, this is a session moment in the first year of treatment:

The patient flew into the room and appeared very excited, talking very fast. "My case conference went great. I got everything I wanted. I couldn't believe it." He kept breaking out into fits of giggling and continued: "All I need is a bit more group work and a bit more work with you and then I'm out of here." I tried in vain to take up his omnipotent stance where he felt that he could lead the clinical team and me this way and that way, wherever he felt he wanted. "No, no", he shouted back, "I just don't care about any of it. I don't care. If I do, I get all stressed up, and then it backfires on me. If I don't care, then no stress, and it all works out—see? Yippee, it's great, I don't give a damn." He then danced around the room, singing.

Only two years into his treatment did Mr C start to consider the possibility that he had problems that needed to be addressed. Here is another session extract one year later from a session that followed on from a further case conference:

"In fact, I'm not well at all but ... I can't be seen to say that to them [the clinical team]. You know the kind of thoughts I'm getting in my mind. And they are all saying how well I am doing. I'm just as mucked up now as I was before—worse, in fact, because I can see it."

In terms of Axis I—Experience of illness and pre-requisites for treatment—here we can see how this young man's experience of being ill and insight is almost entirely lacking upon admission and for much of that first year. He lacks awareness of the severity of his mental symptoms; this is hardly surprising, since he has had to develop a formidable manic repertoire of defences to protect himself from this awareness, which could otherwise feel psychically catastrophic to him. As a result of this, he has no expectations or readiness to receive treatment but attends what is offered. However, this is only with the aim of showing compliance so that he will be "released". He presents an idealized picture of the adverse but familiar social environment outside the hospital setting that he comes from and dismisses the perceived penal, authoritative environment that he has entered, where nurses are known as "screws" and doctors are perceived as being neither proper doctors nor screws but some strange hybrid needing to be placated.

At this early stage of his treatment, Mr C's interpersonal relations (Axis II) are also severely limited. He presents himself as the ward clown who is always happy and joking. He relates to others only in this way, wanting to make everyone laugh, and he is successful to an extent, especially in his relating to other patients who all want to be his friend. This popularity reinforces his clowning around to maintain this popularity and, in particular, as a way of maintaining a distance from anything serious. It is very persuasive, and the clinical team members can be prone to colluding with his humorous style as this enables them to temporarily leave the otherwise difficult and painful working atmosphere they are in. In his presence, one can feel sad that this poor adolescent is so far removed from his real situation and desperate to be liked in this superficial, manic way. These Axis II observations were important to feed back to the clinical team regularly to enable the team members to understand better what Mr C tried to provoke, or create, around him in terms of reactions in others. This understanding could then be used to help the team provide him with a more unified response (Stasch, 2004). Thereby, a more therapeutic attempt to listen and provide containment instead of a mixture of different responses—for example, some collusive, some avoidant, and some too correctional—could be provided.

There are many theoretical approaches to describing mental structure, and Axis IV describes this as the place where identity, character, or personality comes into play. In this system, it is described with six reference points: self-perception, self-regulation, defence, object perception, communication, and attachment. Even though the mental structure is stable over time, it contains dynamic aspects of development that can enable the personality to grow and develop during one's lifetime. A good level of integration is marked by internal and interpersonal regulating functions being available to the patient, independently of external or internal stress.

In terms of Mr C's mental structure, which of course dictates the way Mr C is capable of relating to himself and to others (Axis II), we can see that upon admission he presents with moderate integration of some of these aspects described above. His capacity for self-reflection is limited, and his self-identity is insecure and can fluctuate according to his state of mind, placing him in the moderate level of integration. His capacity to regulate his affects (self-regulation) is impeded, as shown in his near-constant need to present himself as very happy and avoid negative affects at all costs. In the stable environment of the ward within a high-security hospital environment, where acute external stressors are minimized, this remained the case for over a year, and it was well into the second year of treatment before Mr C could allow sad feelings to surface and be tolerated. His main manifest defence mode was aimed at keeping his affects at bay, and he mainly used denial of the manic variety to achieve this, placing him in the moderate level of integration at this stage of his treatment. Less obvious at the start was the degree of splitting and projection required to maintain his happy-go-lucky presentation, to himself as well as to others. His ability to perceive others in all their colours was also impeded and limited his capacity for empathy. He needed to maintain a polarized view of the world where people were idealized or devalued. As long as conflicts were avoided, including interpretations during sessions for which he was not yet ready, he could maintain the idealized image of the other. As soon as a disagreement or contrasting opinion arose—for example, the wish by another patient to view a different television channel, or his therapist making a premature interpretation—then the other became instantly devalued. Mr C's way of communicating with others indicated that he was far away from being able to convey his own thoughts and feelings—which he remained defended against—and also far from being able to take into account the others' thoughts and feelings. Attachment in this context describes the ability to bond with important others, and Mr C's ability to do so was impaired at the start by his limited capacity to perceive the other, as described above. However, despite his dreadful early history and how he presented upon admission, he was, from the start, able to attach himself to important figures, including his therapist, and maintain and develop the rapport. In other words, he was able to gradually develop his (hidden) capacity for object constancy, although the variability of his object relations was restricted.

In the course of his overall treatment plan, in which Mr C continued to have long-term psychotherapy with a consistent therapist and benefited from an ever-stronger therapeutic alliance, the patient made progress, as illustrated in a contrasting description of those three axes several years later. For example, if we return to the scene in seventh year of his treatment described earlier, where the other patient smokes a cigarette outside his new room, which he has been cleaning, it can be seen that this is a patient who experienced something that troubled him, thought about it for a couple of days, and then came to his session and was able to describe the scene, how it left him feeling, and that this feeling had left him puzzled. This is quite a different person from the one who used to fly into the room, sing and dance around, far away from any real feelings about himself and his predicament or what had happened that led to his admission. Here he shows that he is thinking about himself and several others in relation to a situation, which turns out to be unpleasant. He is able to feel angry and confused and hold on to those affects without resorting to an outburst of rage or of manic denial. In terms of Axis IV, he now shows a better level of integration regarding self-perception, self-regulation, more mature defences, better object perception, much improved ability to communicate; attachment to his therapist and important others is relatively stable and secure.

With Axis II in mind, we can see that Mr C's interpersonal relating has also changed remarkably. He is now more flexible in his relating style, able to present himself in different states, including more overtly vulnerable states where he can let the other know he is sad and trust that he will find an appropriate response from the other. If he does not get the hoped-for response, he can accept disappointment provoked by the other without this overwhelming him. Mr C was angry with the patient for putting him on the spot and with the nurses for not believing him. He did not enact his anger or disappointment but was able to hold on to this and bring it to his session.

With Axis I in mind, he has become a patient who is aware that a catastrophe occurred called "killing his mother". For example, he said to me in his seventh year of treatment: "Can you imagine, Doctor Minne, I killed my mother, and I have to live with that fact and that memory all my life. I cannot, and must not, ever get over that, but I know I have to find a way of living with it." At that time, he was also able to empathize with another person, his brother. He said to me in the same session: "One of the things that makes me feel really guilty is that I made my brother lose his mother, and he got nothing out of it. I got all this [waves his hands around indicating the hospital], and he got nothing, and it was not him that killed her." This contrasts with the young man seven years earlier who did not even mention the subject of the killing and wavered between being dissociated from or in manic denial of the tragedy.

In the eighth year of treatment, Mr C experienced for the first time himself coming to a session rather than me going to see him. This involved receiving Home Office permission to attend the Portman Clinic escorted by a nurse, as described earlier. This new phase or promotion was, as previous promotions, exciting and made him anxious. He indicated his anxiety to me by talking very fast, loudly, and jumping on the couch, which he later told me had alarmed him as he thought it was a bed. For a moment he was not sure if he was in my bedsit flat or if the "bed" (couch) was there to seduce him. One of the most obvious areas of progress made by this patient is his capacity to feel different affects, including unpleasant ones, and be able to manage these without gross enactment.

Later on, in the ninth year, Mr C finally received Home Office permission to attend the Portman Clinic unaccompanied. This led to the incident of him returning to his home territory and getting intoxicated with old friends. His conscious reason for going there was that he felt obliged to go back and check that he did not owe anyone anything—that he had been arrested so fast ten years earlier that he had not had time to settle any debts. I considered that he went back to check that he had indeed actually changed, and he was disappointed to see just how quickly regression could arise when he felt demands were too much. In this case, the demand was from me and the clinical team expecting him to manage yet another "promotion": to that of being a responsible person who could be trusted to travel alone. Even though this incident could be seen as quite a worrying development, it also consisted of him telephoning me to let me know where he was and what he had done. In other words, despite his enactment, he retained the capacity to maintain or at least retrieve a part of his mind that knew he was in trouble, and he managed to seek help before the situation escalated. It would be difficult to envision this without the attention placed on treatment-effective therapy and a consistent care provider. This incident was followed by several months of work in sessions around the fact of his "relapse", his loss of permission for unescorted leave, and his own sense of having betrayed himself or having felt betrayed by me. The incident served as a warning to his carers as well as to him that perhaps too much was happening too quickly for him, and we needed to slow the pace of his rehabilitation to eventually living back in the community. Interestingly, one of the striking things Mr C requested during this "post-lapse" period was as follows: "Doctor Minne, could you please let the team know that one session per week is just not enough? I need at least two per week if I am going to be able to get there safely." He recognized that as his external support structure lessened, there was more demand on his internal support structure, and he wanted more "internal" support during this time.

The aim of this type of therapy as part of the overall treatment is to attempt to help the patient to develop knowledge of himself, what he has done, and what kind of mental life he lived that allowed the tragedy to happen. This can only work in the context of support from the clinical team who are regularly informed by the therapist of mental state changes and in the context of physical security, which provides the necessary boundaries before the internal boundaries have formed. With the regular feedback, clinical team members can be alerted to the anticipated patient provocations and offer more unified therapeutic responses, not the unprocessed, mixed, counter-transferential responses that can otherwise arise. This "tuning" of the team could be said to provide the necessary immunization against the contagious symptoms of personality disorders. The communication between the therapist and the clinical team offers the patient a new model of "parenting" where the "parents" communicate thoughtfully about the patient instead of exposing the patient to frightening and perplexing violent actions.

I will now summarize what mental structural changes were monitored and observed to have changed in this patient. The first necessary change that arises in the damaged mental structure is in the area of attachment by offering a stable, balanced person to relate to over a long period of time, enabling the patient to develop object constancy, which he has not had a chance to develop previously through the therapeutic relationship. Further changes in other aspects of structural dimensions then have a chance to germinate. First, in self-perception, the patient develops some curiosity about his new situation, and after many attempts over years trying to get the object to respond in the expected way and, in many instances perceiving this to be the case, he becomes able to take the risk that the object may be different. In the presence of a constant object, albeit one that is still perceived as unpredictable to the patient, he can gradually develop a capacity for self-reflection. Second, after hundreds of occasions identifying the various affects in sessions, the patient becomes aware of these when they arise (externally or internally provoked) and eventually is even able to differentiate between them. Simultaneously, the capacity for object perception evolves with concomitant subject–object differentiation, awareness of the other, and, thereby, the beginning of a capacity for empathy with, much later on in treatment, consequent guilt and remorse. In Mr C's case, feeling able to contact me following his relapse was an achievement that should not go unnoticed. With the improved self- and object perceptions, attachments gradually become less disordered, communication becomes more reciprocal, and the main defence modes, which relate to these other structural dimensions, can mature. Regulation and tolerance of affects can be more internally located and less reliant on external measures. However, it is important to note that at times of stress, when increased demands are placed on the patient, the mental state can regress, and this is when a return to previous functioning, albeit in a modified way, is possible. At these times, patients are prone to minor re-enactments, which can provoke major anxiety in those looking after them. The mental structural changes remain fragile and can shift back to being less integrated. The clinical experience to date with a small group of patients offered long-term psychoanalytic psychotherapy is that the risk of major enactment may be better anticipated and, therefore, prevented or lessened in severity by the detailed psychoanalytic knowledge of the patient, which also provides containment for the patient.

Due to the structural changes that occur, the experience of remorse can arise and is accompanied by a complex mixture of depressed and angry feelings with a psychic longing to return to a state of oblivion. Mr C once said: "It's much worse for me now Doctor, all this thinking and analysing. But I could never go back to how I was before you helped me train the muscles of my mind, even though I'd like to sometimes. Before, if I didn't like something, I'd smash it to pieces. Now, if I don't like something, I start thinking, now why don't I like that? Oh, it's for this or that reason, and so on. By the time I've worked it out, I don't feel like smashing it up any more."

What may have happened to Mr C during this ten-year period if he had not received continuous psychoanalytic psychotherapy? I suspect that at every move down the security chain or "promotion" there would have been a greater risk of enactment that may not have been anticipated and/or contained. This could mean that he may have returned to high security or needed to stay longer in medium security. This would have caused him extreme distress as well as dismay for those caring for him. Furthermore, this would have cost the taxpayer more than the steady progression to the community.

Thinking back to my earlier analogy, it would not occur to commissioners or providers to request or provide time-limited treatments for patients suffering from diabetes or, furthermore, with an expectation of a cure. However, for those patients suffering from "diabetes of the mind", time-limited treatments are the order of the day, often with an unrealistic expectation that a cure be the outcome and an implied criticism when this is not achieved. The importance of attachments, interpersonal relations, and "working through" is neglected within these current treatment systems. Perhaps it is time for us all, treaters and funders, to review the prognostic optimism (or even idealization) in the area of severe mental ill-health and to address seriously the issues of mental health treatments always being about "moving on" to an undefined finishing line. The "cured" patient is then meant to live well in the community. But in fact it is a big achievement for these patients to develop some internal tools that allow them to get consistently better—whereas "cure" appears here to be a term reflecting managerial pressures more than clinical reality. In my view, optimal treatment, good risk management, and being cost-effective is best provided in the context of "knowing" our patients—that is, offering them and/or their clinical teams a continuous psychoanalytic framework.

Acknowledgement

I would like to thank Philip Lurie for his help editing this chapter.

References

APA (1980). *Diagnostic and Statistical Manual of Mental Disorders* (3rd edition). Washington, DC: American Psychiatric Association.

DoH (2009). *The Bradley Report: Lord Bradley's Review of People with Mental Health Problems or Learning Disabilities in the Criminal Justice System.* London: Department of Health. Available at: www.dh.gov.uk/en/Publicationsandstatistics/Publications/PublicationsPolicyAndGuidance/DH_098694

Fallon, P., Blugrass, R., Edwards, B., & Daniels, G. (1999). *The Report of the Committee of Inquiry into the Personality Disorder Unit, Ashworth Special Hospital.* Cmd. 4194-II. London: The Stationery Office.

NICE (2009). *Antisocial Personality Disorder: Full Guideline.* NICE Clinical Guideline 77. London: National Institute for Health and Clinical Excellence. Available at: http://guidance.nice.org.uk/CG77

OPD Task Force (2001). *Operationalized Psychodynamic Diagnostics: Foundations and Manual*. Seattle: Hogrefe & Huber.

Reed, J. (1992). *Review of Mental Health and Social Services for Mentally Disordered Offenders and Others Requiring Similar Services, Vol. 1: Final Summary Report*. Cmd. 2088. London: HMSO.

Salekin, R. (2002). Psychopathy and therapeutic pessimism: Clinical lore or clinical reality. *Clinical Psychology Review, 22*: 79–112.

Stasch, M. (2004). *Interpersonal Tuning in Inpatient Psychotherapy: A Clinical Approach Based on the Operationalized Psychodynamic Diagnostics (OPD)*. Paper presented at the 34th Annual Meeting of the Society for Psychotherapy Research, Weimar, Germany.

Tilt, R., Perry, B., Martin, C., Maguire, N., & Preston, M. (2000). *Report of the Review of Security at the High Security Hospitals*. London: Department of Health.

Warren, F. (2003). *Review of Treatments for Severe Personality Disorder*. Home Office online report. Available at: www.floridatac.org/files/document/rdsolr3003.pdf

WHO (1992). *International Statistical Classification of Diseases and Related Health Problems* (10th revision, ICD-10). Geneva: World Health Organization.

CHAPTER SEVEN

Picking up a log from both ends: couple work in the Tavistock tradition

Joanna Rosenthall

> The idea of a couple coming together to produce a child is central in our psychic life, whether we aspire to it, object to it, realise we are produced by it, deny it, relish it, or hate it.
>
> Ron Britton (1989, p. xi)

The history of "Tavistock" couple work started in the period following the Second World War. The new leadership at the Tavistock wanted to establish the clinic's place in the newly established NHS, which involved major reorganization. According to Henry Dicks, the changes evoked resistance from the old guard, who felt that "playing with innovations like group therapy and other 'perversions' of Freud's technique was a very dangerous 'deviationism'" (1970, p. 6).

One of these "perversions" was psychoanalytically informed couple work, which was split between two organizations: the Marital Unit in the Tavistock Clinic, which had opted into the NHS, headed by Henry Dicks, and another grouping emerging from the Family Welfare Association, called the Family Discussion Bureau, later the Institute of Marital Studies, now the Tavistock Centre for Couple Relationships (TCCR). While the present-day Couples Unit in the

Tavistock and Portman NHS Trust and the TCCR are separate bodies situated in different organizational contexts, they both have their roots in the "Tavistock Family" and share the philosophy of developing clinical work with couples using a psychoanalytic approach.

From social to psychological marriage

After the Second World War, health professionals were confronted with increasing numbers of "broken homes". A Royal Commission on Marriage and Divorce report published in 1956 expressed concern about the rate of marriage breakdown, and there was fear that it was reaching epidemic proportions, which might explain why Dicks asked whether marital strife was "a kind of substitute psychiatric illness" (1967, p. 4).

After this period, the social context changed, including the role and aspiration of women, and, significantly, the divorce rate soared until the mid-1990s, when nearly 50% of marriages ended in divorce. It is worth remembering that the civil registration of marriages dates back only to 1836; the formal institution of marriage can therefore be seen as being the product of a relatively recent historical cycle that, perhaps not surprisingly, has been through its own phases of upheaval and change.

During the 1950s and 1960s the study of marriage became the project of both the Tavistock Clinic and the Institute of Marital Studies (IMS). Both organizations viewed marriage and the couple relationship as the foundation of adult mental health as well as a site of considerable disturbance: the correlation between "couple health" and child development is now well established (Lewis, Beavers, Gossett, & Phillips, 1976; Pape Cowan & Cowan, 1997). After the 1960s, the main theoretical and clinical developments took place within the IMS/TCCR; there was a prolific output of publications, action research projects, innovations in technique, and applications of psychoanalytic ideas that contributed to a national debate about the nature of marriage and the social policy to support it (Clulow & Mattinson, 1989; Fisher, 1999; Fisher & Ruszczynski, 1995; Grier, 2005; Mattinson & Sinclair, 1979; Ruszczynski, 1993).

The preoccupation with marriage as social or psychological fluctuates depending on the contemporary anxiety about the perceived quality of social cohesion. In recent years there has been what amounts to "moral" panic about rising divorce rates, falling marriage rates, and a growing tendency for cohabitation and child-rearing outside marriage. Social and economic forces have changed the meaning and, to an extent, the nature of marriage. To reflect this, both organizations changed their names, replacing "marital" with "couple", implicitly recognizing same-sex as well as heterosexual relationships and the significance of considering a psychological state of "marriage" rather than the formal institution.

The couple as patient

From the outset the Marital Unit wanted to prioritize the psychodynamics of relationships; in the words of Dr Donnan, one of the psychiatrists at the time:

> Marriage is one of the largest of human relationships, and to attempt to assess and deal with the difficulties of one partner without coming to know something of the other, and without a regard to the relationship between them, is like trying to lift a log by one end only. [Dicks, 1967, p. 2]

In the early days, each partner had a separate clinician each of whom met to discuss the work. In the 1960s, influenced by group therapy, the partners were seen together. This innovation had an enormous impact because instead of hearing reports about difficulties, the clinician was able to have a unique experience of the couple in the consulting room. Many of the subsequent developments came out of this change, and currently most couples are seen conjointly. This work has since been influenced by the theoretical and clinical contributions of many (especially the work of Balint, 1959; Bion, 1959; Klein, 1946; Winnicott, 1965; and, more recently, Britton, 1989; Kohon, 1999; Steiner, 1993).

In aim, working with a couple differs little from working with an individual, except that the focus is on the couple as the patient, not on the two partners as individuals. With that at the forefront, it is important to be aware of each individual's state of mind, their central preoccupations, particularly the shared ones, the nature of the transference and the countertransference, the symbolic meaning of the material, and their individual and shared histories. In this chapter, I have chosen to highlight two areas of shared unconscious activity—the projective system and the shared unconscious phantasy—and show how they can provide us with a rough but meaningful "couple geography" of shared unconscious dynamics.

The projective system and partner choice

Underpinning the work is the image of the couple and the fulfilment associated with it, rooted in the earliest of all relationships—that is to say, the residual memory of the state of reverie between mother and infant.

Falling in love is one of the most powerful experiences of the unconscious at work but, like all unconscious processes, is out of reach and difficult to understand. Partners appear to "choose" each other on the basis of finding someone who will receive one's own repudiated projections. The concept of projective identification helps understanding, in that each partner is a willing recipient of the other's projections—both unwanted and also wanted idealized parts. In short, a couple relationship can be conceived of as "a mutual transference relationship" (Ruszczynski, 1993). An everyday colloquialism, "opposites attract", captures this more simply.

Initially, each person is relieved of unmanageable parts of his or her own experience, leading to a wonderful feeling of acceptance and love. Freud himself likened it to delusion (1930a, p. 56), and without doubt there is a repudiation of reality. Each partner not only receives idealized representations that initially are welcome, but also "gets rid of" unwanted parts of themselves; there is probably a shared phantasy that these difficult parts of the self need never be faced again, which might explain the experience of elation.

Falling in love has a parallel with the passionate first love between mother and baby. There continues to be a longing for a primitive state of fusion, where all needs are taken care of and no frustration is experienced. Falling in love can temporarily "provide it". The desire for the ideal, and the phantasy that it exists, is a primitive and powerful psychological force that very often drives the early stages of a relationship.

This produces a painful paradox: the individuals are now in close daily contact with the realities of mutual projective identification, including those very aspects of themselves that they can least manage. The repudiated parts, now located in the other, cannot be forgotten, as they tend to be frequently enacted in everyday life, albeit now experienced as residing in the other and not within the self. When large amounts of the personality are projected in this way, each partner's behaviour is affected, often being nudged into extreme opposites. They tend to portray themselves and experience the other in stereotypical ways—for example, "she's the emotional one and he's the angry one"—and, when they are under the sway of each other's projections, are more likely to get stuck in vicious-circle patterns of relating. It is very often this kind of experience that brings a couple into treatment.

McDougall provides a useful parallel when she describes individuals who cannot manage to apprehend the facts and details of their lives and resort to externalizing inner conflicts by various means—for example, by relying on substances like drugs or food, or else on other people. She describes a "transitional theatre" in which the individual plays a part and chooses others to enact parts that cannot be borne psychically. The wish behind such complicated dramas is to "try and make sense of what the small child of the past, who is still writing the scripts, found too confusing to understand" (McDougall, 1986, p. 65). These individuals, instead of forming symptoms, are dominated by "action symptoms", which perform a similar function, binding together psychic experiences that cannot be borne or known about. In a couple both partners derive relief from externalizing unresolved mental pain. At the same time, this defensive strategy tends to mean that the relationship can only take place in a restricted zone, which may look deeply unhappy, even hate-filled to the observer. The couples, too, often come and express their incredulity that things are so awful, they just can't understand why they are still together.

In a relationship that supports each partner's development, each partner gradually takes back projections into the self and develops a greater capacity to tolerate emotional pain, resulting in a deeper and broader emotional repertoire and a greater ability to face the realities of life. Problems in a relationship tend to arise when the need to repudiate parts of the self is stronger than the urge to develop and mature. In most couple relationships these defensive needs and developmental hopes are in a continual state of tension.

Idealization helps partners to take the enormous step of choosing a life partner. However, the process of individual maturation involves managing more and more aspects of one's self within the boundary of one's own mind, with a decreasing need to project parts of the self into others. From this perspective, the couple relationship is there to support an individual process of development. Each partner can be thought of as pursuing a journey, a kind of "psychic orienteering" (Rosenthall, 2007)—a process of discovering his or her own identity both as an individual and in relation to the other. The main tasks are, broadly: managing psychological separation, tolerating frustration, relinquishing a position of narcissism, and bearing pain and disillusionment. The couple relationship can support or hinder these tasks. A more flexible interaction allows each partner to explore the conflicts involved in the need for individuation and also for intimacy. It is important to recognize that these struggles are lifelong, and have to be "reworked, at each stage of development and with each major addition to experience or knowledge" (Britton, 1992, p. 38).

Couples coming for help often arrive in a state of confusion, bordering on chaos, feeling helpless, stuck in a world where they are experiencing the other's repeated provocation or even hate-filled attacks. An attack provokes further retaliation, which sets up a vicious circle. Mutual projection results in utter confusion about what belongs to whom. Before too long, awareness of the vulnerable self and the vulnerable other is out of reach. At the extreme end of this, both partners are lost in a maze of projections that Morgan (1995) has called a "projective gridlock".

One husband seen in the unit recently described this predicament rather well, saying that he felt they were coming with over 300 different problems, all of which they disagreed on, and he didn't know how to know where to start. They had already seen another therapist, and when they left her, he felt they had spent the time sharing some of these problems, showing her how many they had. Not only did he still feel as lost as he had at the start, but he also felt exposed, humiliated, and in despair about whether they could ever find help.

Shared unconscious phantasies and shared defences

Britton (1989) has described the maturational process through the lens of the Oedipus complex, highlighting the significance of the infant's relationship not only to each parent separately, but also to the parental couple as a couple. Melanie Klein (1928) discovered that the individual does not just internalize the actual parents, but the internal picture of them is coloured by projections and introjections. A potent application of this idea is that the nature of the couples' relationship is unconsciously determined by the nature of the partners' relationships to their parents, imbued as they are with their own projections, internalized and then re-enacted in their internal and external object relationships (Ruszczynski, 1993).

Feldman (1999) points out how the patient's dilemmas (he also highlights oedipal dilemmas) are brought into an analysis, often in a way that draws the analyst into a re-enactment of the situation that was originally the child's. Similarly, partners in a couple unconsciously nudge and pressurize each other into re-enactments of their "unconscious internal couple" and as-yet unresolved oedipal dramas.

Forming a couple, each partner comes unconsciously armed with a complex picture of what a couple looks like—a kind of layered template for an intimate adult relationship—but the partners individually also seem to have an unconscious capacity to recognize something shared in the other's internal couple picture. It is likely that these factors create a resonance, which not only seems to contribute towards the "draw" that the individuals feel but also informs the nature of the link between them. After some time in therapy it should be possible to start elaborating the nature of the couple's shared unconscious phantasies, which provides an opportunity to explore the gap between phantasy and reality. This way of understanding shared unconscious phantasies implies that not only do partners share styles of relating, but they also join together in shared defensive structures to avoid disavowed and unbearable internal experiences.

The challenge in working with couples is to bear in mind everything we have learnt as psychoanalytic practitioners and apply this to the system that the two people create—the patient is the couple—so not only do we have the internal situation of each individual, but we also have the relationship between them, which is being enacted in the room. Joseph (1985) endorses Klein's (1952) formulation of the "total situation" that a patient brings into the psychoanalytic relationship. This means that reports about everyday life, stories, the atmosphere in the room, the clinician's own feelings, are all clues to understanding the situation of an individual and, similarly, a couple. However, when there are two people in the room and hence a profusion of material, focusing on certain elements is essential: the relationship itself, the system that the couple create, becomes the focus of understanding.

Couples have a story

Many couples come without a meaningful "narrative". This narrative, which involves not just memories of experiences but some capacity for thinking about themselves and linking them up into what amounts to a personal story, is a crucial part of the development of personal identity. People who are cut off from their past not only seem unreachable and thin, but they also speak of things in a current way as if they have no resonance in the past or with other people. Wollheim (1984) described them as having "broken the thread of life", and he has shown that the thread of life is at the core of personal identity and the person's sense of inner unity.

It is part of the clinical task to discover and put into words a meaningful and coherent story—one that may not be linear but, rather, includes conscious and unconscious elements of each partner's experience as well as the experience of their relationship. In a brief context, one cannot hope to piece together much of this narrative, but even to start conveys that it is possible to discover meaning. This process has an important impact on the couple, serving an integrative and developmental function. Any change in this direction affects the way the partners function together and, perhaps especially in a brief encounter, might whet their appetites for more.

Working with the transference

Very often the partners are consciously aware that they are helplessly caught in a powerful repetition, and they may even laugh at themselves wryly: "I didn't want to be like my parents, but that's exactly what we are. . . ." Two things are important about this: first, they are unable to describe the situation more exactly, and, second, they tend to blame each other so they cannot see, and often don't want to recognize, their own contribution to this dilemma. Keeping the transference as the focus of the thinking helps to piece together a meaningful narrative. Historically, in couple work the transference was considered only necessary to engage with when the transference itself was preventing change. However, in undertaking brief work with couples more recently, I have found it important to keep the transference as a focus of thinking because it illuminates and provides a meaningful relational narrative. It also usefully intensifies the therapeutic experience, which has important consequences in time-limited work.

In order to be aware and alive to the transference relationship, the therapist needs to be available as early in the encounter as possible for a lively emotional engagement. The clinical focus aims to move between the relationship between the partners and the relationship between the couple and the clinician.

If the therapist is able to describe the nature of the relationship between him/herself and the couple, it tends to be easier to explore. It is more bearable to hear and acknowledge something they have done to the therapist than something they have done to each other, which is already an arena of blame and counterattack. In addition, when the therapist describes the way they are trying to dominate or bully, it is possible to do it gently and with respect, so that they can have the experience that their attacks are not damaging but can be thought about and understood. After this kind of exploration, there is often a natural progression for the couple to show interest in how this reflects what they are also doing with each other, which, in turn, often evokes links with the past. When the focus of the exploration is the interaction itself and not one or other of the individuals, this in itself can challenge the atmosphere of blame, which allows further exploration into what unconscious element they are protecting by behaving in this way.

A brief couple therapy

Sara and Ben, a couple in their early forties, came for therapy in a crisis. They jointly conveyed an atmosphere of helpless despair, and I quickly felt mobilized into wanting to help them.

> Ben repeated many times that he saw no option but to leave because he was convinced that his wife not only didn't love him, but that she didn't like him either. He appeared to communicate in a rather naïve and passive way that he just wanted to be close to her and he also wanted to have sex. The reality was that he felt constantly criticized and made to feel no good, and he couldn't

bear the thought of spending the rest of his life in this desolate relationship.

Sara agreed, she did criticize him a lot, but that was because he was so insensitive, clumsy, and, worst of all, he left all their family problems up to her. She wasn't sure she did want sex because her husband fell far short of what she wanted a husband to be, and she conveyed a crushing sense of disappointment and anger.

The couple were prompted to come for therapy because their youngest, a son of 16, had made a serious suicidal gesture. They were understandably extremely anxious about leaving him alone, and he was the source of a lot of their arguing. Having been seen as parents in an adolescent unit, where he was a patient in his own right, there was recognition that they also needed help as a couple, and they were referred to the Couples Unit.

Sara was in a very close, merged relationship with her son. It seemed significant that in their house the son's bedroom was just above the living area and below their bedroom, so when they were downstairs they felt they couldn't speak privately or row because he could hear them in his room, and they couldn't have sex because he would hear them below in his bedroom. From his central position, he was unable to live his own life at all, and yet he was ruling the family and significantly interfering with the parental couple's capacity to be a couple.

A lot of the work in the initial period was focused on the way the mother–son pairing was at the centre of the family while Ben was on the edge, left out as a husband and as a father, as if he were a resentful child. I saw a pattern where Sara berated Ben for not being enough of a reliable parent, so that she could loosen her grip and at least "have a day off"; Ben would weakly attempt to defend himself but would soon collapse into an unreachable silence where it was difficult to tell what he was thinking or feeling. He reported that he did make attempts to be in touch with his son, but he was usually spurned; he would then retreat into a position of "I've done all I can, now look, he's rejected me . . .". All of them, including himself, apparently saw him as weak and useless.

This scenario had an obvious oedipal flavour in which the most potent "hot" relationship was that between mother and son. Sara overtly wanted her husband to relieve her of her terrible burden of having a worrying son, and of the bleakness and flatness in her life. Yet unconsciously she seemed to cling tenaciously to this state of affairs, partly because this was the only relationship in her life where she felt loved and special.

Ben was a man who was unsure about his thoughts and feelings and had even greater difficulty putting them into words. He was passive, as if in hiding, unable to represent himself, waiting for her to take charge, and frequently misunderstanding her feelings as well. It was possible to hear the anger in his voice, but it tended to come out compromised and a bit wooden. She complained that they couldn't get close because he "wasn't there", whereas he felt rejected sexually and desperately longed to be loved in a physical way. They were left with no way of making an intimate connection, stuck in a dynamic repeated constantly where she felt she had no husband—there was no couple because she had to manage everything alone, leaving Ben feeling a weak and useless failure, a bit like a rejected child.

When partners have not negotiated their own oedipal conflicts, it is common to see a relationship in which each is attempting to nudge the other into a mother–child pairing. They want to be held, understood, and cared for by the other, sometimes even feeling that none of it should have to be put into words. From what I could see, Sara and Ben were stuck in their own particular version of this. Each of them was seeking from the other the emotional containment that had been lacking in their early experience. This created a distorted interaction in which each became disappointed and resentful, because they didn't find the loving parent they longed for, but, instead, found someone who was either rejecting or making "unfair" demands of them. It goes without saying that there was no space left and perhaps no capacity in this arena for an adult sexual relationship, which was devastating for them both and catastrophic for their son.

Family histories

Ben and Sara were both the youngest in large families, and they shared a terrible feeling that they were unwanted: their mothers already had enough on their plates, and there wasn't really room for another. In addition, they both had parents who were very unhappily married, either openly rowing or caught in cold silences. In both families, everyone had been under a harsh regime, with no space allowed for discussing feelings or vulnerability, and neither of them could remember any kindness being shown. Sara wept in one session when she told me she wasn't sure if she ever really wanted sex, she didn't think she knew what love was, she didn't remember ever being held or cuddled as a child, and I was left with the impression that she experienced sex as someone uncaringly and clumsily crashing into her. It also seemed important that she highlighted having a cold, critical mother, whereas he felt dominated by a harsh, judgmental father. Arising from these experiences, they seemed to share a conviction that no one would be interested in them, as well as a conviction that if there was contact, it would involve one person dominating or harshly judging the other—a picture that provides a rudimentary outline of an important phantasy that they shared.

In one of the early sessions, a vivid picture of their shared unconscious relationship emerged. Sara started the session noticing that the chairs they were sitting on were closer together than usual, which made her anxious because it gave her the feeling that I had moved them on purpose, so that they would have to get closer, whether they liked it or not.

Ben was unusually animated, telling me how they weren't good together: they couldn't agree on anything or do anything together, they niggled at each other all the time, she couldn't even cross the road with him. The other day they were crossing the road and a big lorry was coming and he went in one direction to go in front of it. She took a different direction with their son, crossing the road, but behind the lorry. Why couldn't she hold his hand and let him lead her over the road? He sounded aggrieved by this.

She went on to say that she also felt the need for something to change. She was caring for their son and doing most of the domestic chores as well; it was all too much, and he just didn't seem able to see that.

They alerted me in this session to their shared conviction that any contact involved "forcing", confirmed by her belief that I had moved the chairs: I was trying to change them by applying pressure, and the way I was doing this was to change something in the external world. They were showing me that they were unable to see each other as separate people, and they believed I too didn't see them as separate from myself. It seemed to them as if I felt that they were out of my reach, so I had to force them to do what I wanted, just as they too felt out of each other's reach and therefore had to find other ways of applying pressure to try to get what they wanted. Using this material I was able to connect up their experience of me in the transference and the way it appeared to be mirrored in their relationship with each other.

This material also hints at some of the shared underlying phantasies that made coupling so terrifying, as if it could lead to death. The road-crossing story implies that they can't take the risk to join up, but neither can they operate separately, so they defensively try to inhabit a limbo world where they keep things static and nothing much can happen: they don't feel nourished and there is a lot of suffering, but at least they are "safe".

While she complained on the one hand, Sara's mind seemed to be taken over by a narcissistic illusion that she could manage alone, that she didn't really need Ben, because she was "right" and he was "wrong", even though this left her very resentful and isolated. When he held out a hand, she didn't take it because she didn't trust him. When he offered her things, sometimes they were superficial and clumsy, but sometimes they were solid and valuable; she, however, tended to dismiss everything he offered as if it was all useless. If she didn't take anything, she could remain in a world of her own making, where she was protected from knowing about her own dependence as well as the rewarding/disappointing mix in any adult couple relationship.

Ben too was stuck in masochistic passivity where he offered his hand, but in his mind he didn't have to do any work to join up with her and form a team. By telling me about this scene, they were showing me that, fuelled by unconscious phantasies, they had a shared conviction that if they tried to join up and be a team/couple, they would be pulling in opposite directions, and something very dangerous might happen—they could die. This left them with an unconscious terror that making contact was too dangerous, but equally if they went their separate ways, they would be left alone. He was desolate and resentful, while she was overburdened and angry, so separately, too, there was deep dissatisfaction and danger of a different kind. This dilemma has been eloquently and vividly described as a universal, primitive dilemma for us all in Glasser's (1979) description of the core complex.

All of this became apparent to me not only through their material, but also in the transference relationship. When I intervened, I sensed that they felt intensely about me, as if they had never experienced this kind of contact before. I sensed that they felt rescued, but it was hard for them to pick anything up and take it forward, so it could feel when I spoke as if I was pronouncing things for them and as if I was a rescuer.

Over the first few months, it gradually dawned on me that not only did the sessions tend to start in the same way, with them apparently needing reassurance and coaxing to come alive a little and share something of their thoughts or experience, but, in addition, there was a sense that nothing had changed and maybe nothing could change. They looked as if they were interested and listening during the sessions, but in fact many of the sessions felt as if we were back to square one, starting again from the very beginning, as if they had retained nothing. I wondered if in fact they had taken anything in from me at all.

It was a relief when I finally put this into words. Sara laughed: she immediately understood and talked movingly and with a new freshness and greater trust about how hard it was to keep these new thoughts in her mind; they evaporated at the door ... challenged everything she knew ... turned things upside down. ... Even though she was acknowledging that it made sense, she was engaged and willing to work, it felt extremely difficult to hold on to any thoughts outside the room. Ben, however seemed not to understand; when I pursued him, it didn't work either, because he withdrew and seemed further away than ever.

I now had an uneven and uncomfortable situation in which Sara seemed more willing or more able to think than Ben did. Whenever I tried to reach him, and however kindly, he seemed unable to respond. He often heard things as criticisms, and attempts to explore this seemed to make it worse. At first I thought he might not be capable of thinking, then I realized that I had been recruited to enact a cold, despairing, perhaps even impatient, parent who has given up on him as if he were second-rate, whereas Sara had become the favoured child who can develop and be rewarding.

We continued in this frustrating way for some months. Then a breakthrough came after they told me, in passing, about a row they'd had. They were reluctant to share it, but intuition told me that there was some hidden life in this story. In turned out to be about how a big crack had developed in their living-room wall and how they had left it for months, unable to resolve a fight between them about the cause, and therefore what the solution should be. It became clear that they had had several major rows, both convinced they were right and the other was wrong, and any discussion became a fight for survival as only one of them was "right" and the other would be humiliated—habitually Ben's position.

Exploring this with me and being able to bear the idea that they were both longing to be heard, understood, and taken into account allowed them to loosen their grip on certainties and make a little more space for each other. I think they were interested by the ideas I offered them—a shared conviction (unconscious phantasy) that there was only room for one of them, only one idea was of value, which meant they were constantly having life-and-death fights and also that they shared a feeling that something was wrong inside—"cracked and not whole". There was a new sense of liveliness in the room, and soon after this they spent a weekend together moving their son into the top bedroom that they had occupied and themselves moving into his, thereby freeing themselves up in the living room and the bedroom. A space for the couple was emerging.

Gradually they opened up a little more, and in one session they shared what things had been like at the start. Neither of them could articulate what had drawn them to the other. After some difficulty, he managed to relay a very painful story of how soon after they'd started a relationship, she told him she was going away for a short break to see another man. When she returned, this wasn't discussed. He felt he had been in a very dark place but struggled now to put words to his pain, his rage, and his enormous sense of an internal lack. She couldn't really explain her cruelty, but it enabled all of us to see that right at the start this painful dynamic had been part of what they shared and was probably also part of what drew them to each other. It was as if they were both preoccupied with feeling not special and unlovable, and she had cruelly enacted it with him, projecting her own second-rate, unloveable qualities into him as if she could be freed of them while he had a "double dose". Here the sadomasochism was performing a defensive purpose, while the relationship continued to hold the promise of something deeper and more fulfilling. It was probably also true that he projected the angry, critical qualities into her so that he was apparently devoid of aggression while she was brimming over with it.

From this material I was able to connect this version of a relationship to the one they had with me, as well as the one they had together. Not only did they cruelly rise above each other and fight for the higher position, but they unconsciously did the same to me when they ignored what I offered, giving me the experience of starting from the beginning at each session. I now understood that when I offered them interpretations, I too was experienced as interrogating and humiliating them as "second-rate". They were unaware of this but lived it by dropping what I said at the door and refusing to take it in. I, in turn, felt frustrated and puzzled, tempted to either coldly repeat interpretations or to think of them as a hopeless case—people who could never use the help to change. Effectively, they were saying to me, "what you say is no good, it doesn't help, you are second rate, not us", and I was effectively retaliating either with barren repetitions or by giving up hope. Only as things started to shift did I more fully realize that we had been stuck, doomed in each session to repeatedly start again from the very beginning.

After some exploration of all of this, Sara joined in to say that what I had been describing was true, and it frequently happened between the two of them as well, she recognized it. It was noticeable to me that during this discussion, both of them seemed alive and awake, providing more and more material for how they frequently re-enacted similar sorts of scenes with each other and with their son and they even brought memories from their own childhoods, which deepened the picture and gave them the chance to feel more fully known and understood.

It seemed that a lot of the discussions in their present family and their families of origin had felt like interrogations, Sara confirmed this, saying it was like second nature, she had to do it because Ben often got it wrong.

This gave me the opportunity to start to talk about how they shared a picture of a relationship in which there was a harsh domineering figure and a weak, speechless child. When I was the harsh figure, they became like passive children, waiting for me to breathe life into them. They felt angry or hurt but couldn't share it with me out of fear that I would not be interested or I would retaliate and go cold on them. When they were alone together, her inclination was to take up the controlling, forceful, domineering figure who asks interrogating questions and is always right, while he became the resentful, frozen child. As this was explored, Ben became more lively and genuinely interested, and eventually I was able to raise the idea of how they might both be full of sensitive areas and could easily feel they were being trampled over; the way they related probably meant that their tender areas were ignored.

At this point in the therapy it felt as if we had weathered something that had never been faced by them before. My relationship with each of them felt deeper and more meaningful, and they too seemed a little freer; there was more warmth and more hope between them.

Steiner (2008, p. 70) has described how when the analyst is experienced as acting independently, outside the patient's control, this can promote a situation in which the patient might bear the independence of the analyst and mourn the loss of what he calls "the possessive relationship", and a degree of separateness is achieved, disowned parts of the self are regained, and the individual is enriched. I have described some elements of this. Over time, not only did Sara and Ben let go of me as a cruel dominator, but they also loosened this structure with each other.

Conclusion

The couple relationship is of central importance across the whole life span. It is perplexing that so little attention is given to it clinically, in spite of the fact that the nature of the couple relationship impacts on both the quality of parenting and the mental health of adult individuals, to say nothing of its contribution to the formation of citizens.

As far as parenting work goes, a combination of factors appears to have led to an emphasis on work with the primary carer (usually the mother), leaving the couple relationship not sufficiently attended to. This trend is apparent throughout child services, although NICE guidelines recognize that:

> Family risk factors for depression in children and adolescents include parent–child conflict, parental discord, divorce and sepa- ration, parental death, parental mental illness and parental sub- stance misuse. . . . The risk is thought not to lie in the variable per se but in its effects on attitudes, behaviour and relationships within the family. [NICE, 2004, pp. 62–63]

Many couples who seek help would never present themselves as individual patients. This is because the couple relationship itself can act as a structure, holding and supporting troubled individuals. Help for adult couple relationships can enhance the mutual support vulnerable individuals provide for each other. NICE guidelines recognize this also, recommending that couple-focused therapy should be considered for patients with depression who have a regular partner and who have not benefited from a brief intervention (NICE, 2009, p. 25). This conclusion was based on research that found that couple therapy worked better than antidepressants in the treatment of adult depression (Leff et al., 2000).

All of this thinking points to the necessity and value of develop- ing a more inclusive view of the couple relationship in mental health provision for individuals of all ages. Is its present omission fuelled by familiarity with the couple or even by an unresolved oedipal terror of "meddling" in an area that seems sacrosanct and ultimately private? Psychoanalysis shows the need to straddle both the "order" of theory and the muddle of emotional experience; in Enid Balint's words, we too need to be able to "tolerate the absence of a consistent story for a time and use the muddle" (1993, p. 166).

> For one human being to love another: that is perhaps the most dif- ficult of our tasks; the ultimate, the last test and proof, the work for which all other work is but preparation. [Rainer Maria Rilke][1]

Note

1. From *Letters to a Young Poet*, written between 1903 and 1908 to a student, Franz Kappus, who had sent Rilke his poems for evaluation. The quotation is from Letter Seven, dated 14 May 1904.

References

Balint, E. (1993). *Before I Was I: Psychoanalysis and the Imagination. Collected Papers of Enid Balint*, ed. J. Mitchell & M. Parsons. London: Free Association Books.

Balint, M. (1959). *Thrills and Regressions*. London: Hogarth Press.

Bion, W. R. (1959). Attacks on linking. *International Journal of Psychoanalysis, 40*: 308–315. Also in: *Second Thoughts*. London: Karnac, 1984.

Britton, R. (1989). The missing link: Parental sexuality in the Oedipus complex. In: J. Steiner (Ed.), *The Oedipus Complex Today: Clinical Implications* (pp. 83–101). London: Karnac.

Britton, R. (1992). The Oedipus situation and the depressive position. In: R. Anderson (Ed.), *Clinical Lectures on Klein and Bion* (pp. 34–45). London: Routledge.

Clulow, C. F., & Mattinson, J. (1989). *Marriage Inside Out*. Harmondsworth: Penguin.

Dicks, H. V. (1967). *Marital Tensions: Clinical Studies towards a Psychological Theory of Interaction*. London: Routledge & Kegan Paul.

Dicks, H. V. (1970). *Fifty Years of the Tavistock Clinic*. London: Routledge & Kegan Paul.

Feldman, M. (1999). The Oedipus complex: Manifestations in the inner world and the therapeutic situation. In: J. Steiner (Ed.), *The Oedipus Complex Today: Clinical Implications*. London: Karnac.

Fisher, J. (1999). *The Uninvited Guest: Emerging from Narcissism towards Marriage*. London: Karnac.

Fisher, J., & Ruszczynski, S. (Eds.) (1995). *Intrusion and Intimacy in the Couple Relationship*. London: Karnac.

Freud, S. (1930a). *Civilization and Its Discontents. Standard Edition, 21*.

Glasser, M. (1979). Aggression and sadism in the perversions. In: I. Rosen (Ed.), *Sexual Deviation*. Oxford: Oxford University Press.

Grier, F. (Ed.) (2005). *Oedipus and the Couple*. London: Karnac.

Joseph, B. (1985). Transference: The total situation. *International Journal of Psychoanalysis, 66*: 447–454.

Klein, M. (1928). Early stages of the Oedipus conflict. In: *Love, Guilt and Reparation and Other Works* (pp. 186–198). London: Hogarth Press, 1975.

Klein, M. (1946). Notes on some schizoid mechanisms. In: *Envy and Gratitude and Other Works* (pp. 1–25). London: Hogarth Press, 1975.

Klein, M. (1952). The origins of transference. In: *Envy and Gratitude and Other Works* (pp. 48–56). London: Hogarth Press, 1975.

Kohon, G. (1999). *No Lost Certainties to Be Recovered*. London: Karnac.

Leff, J., Vearnals, S., Wolff, G., Alexander, B., Chisolm, D., Everitt, B., et al. (2000). Randomised controlled trial of antidepressants versus couple therapy in the treatment and maintenance of people with depression living with a partner: Clinical outcome and costs. *British Journal of Psychiatry, 177*: 95–100.

Lewis, J., Beavers, W., Gossett, J., & Phillips, V. (1976). *No Single Thread: Psychological Health in Family Systems*. New York: Brunner/Mazel.

Mattinson, J., & Sinclair, I. (1979). *Mate and Stalemate*. Oxford: Blackwell.

McDougall, J. (1986). *Theatres of the Mind*. London: Free Association Books.

Morgan, M. (1995). The projective gridlock: A form of projective identification in couple relationships. In: S. Ruszczynski & J. Fisher (Eds.), *Intrusiveness and Intimacy in the Couple*. London: Karnac.

NICE (2004). *CG28: Depression in Children and Young Adults*. London: National Institute for Health and Clinical Excellence. Available at: www.nice.org.uk

NICE (2009). *CG91: Depression in Adults with a Chronic Physical Health Problem: Nice Guidelines*. London: National Institute for Health and Clinical Excellence. Available at: www.nice.org.uk

Pape Cowan, C., & Cowan, P. (1997). Working with couples during stressful transitions. In: S. Dreman (Ed.), *The Family on the Threshold of the 21st Century: Trends and Implications*. Mahwah, NJ: Lawrence Erlbaum Associates.

Rosenthall, J. (2007). Sharing a heart: The dilemma of a fused couple. *British Journal of Psychotherapy, 23*: 411–429.

Royal Commission on Marriage and Divorce (1956). *Report of the Royal Commission on Marriage and Divorce*. Cmd. 9678. London: HMSO.

Ruszczynski, S. (1993). Thinking about and working with couples. In: S. Ruszczynski (Ed.), *Psychotherapy with Couples*. London: Karnac.

Steiner, J. (1993). *Psychic Retreats*. London: Routledge.

Steiner, J. (Ed.) (2008). *Rosenfeld in Retrospect: Essays on His Clinical Influence*. London: Routledge.

Winnicott, D. W. (1965). *The Maturational Processes and the Facilitating Environment*. London: Karnac, 1990.

Wollheim, R. (1984). *The Thread of Life*. Cambridge: Press Syndicate of the University of Cambridge.

INNOVATIONS IN
ADULT MENTAL HEALTH CARE

Introduction

Alessandra Lemma

This book provides a snapshot of an institution the reputation of which as a provider of high-quality mental health care and training is undisputed, and yet its survival in its current form as a relatively small Mental Health Trust is uncertain. The anxiety this uncertainty generates has spurred creative developments. The contributors to Part III illustrate an impressive capacity to adapt to new demands and social realities that challenge the limits of any one therapeutic modality or mode of service delivery. Inevitably, there are many services that could not be included due to the constraints of space, but the contributions reflect a representative range of applications rooted in a broadly defined psychoanalytic tradition. They give a flavour of applications across the age range, which are delivered in different contexts.

This work deserves celebration, not least because such developments, which often rely on integrating different ways of working, have been hard won: living under one roof, as it were, does not imply that we all share the same point of view or that our differences are managed with the generosity and openness of mind that we aspire to. Behind every developmental process there are inevitable regressions too: there are stalemates and tensions that are part of organizational life and that are impossible to work through once and for all; rather, they need to be worked on and reworked repeatedly because their nature is that they are not resolvable in any absolute sense: they are part of group life.

Adaptations of the psychoanalytic model of intensive psychotherapy/analysis may understandably mobilize a range of anxieties. Such adaptations seem to arouse concern that psychoanalysis will be damaged by the intrusion of other ways of theorizing, thinking, and practising. Integration and adaptation may be presented as development but experienced as undermining (Lemma & Johnston, 2010). For example, the *application* of psychoanalytic theory and techniques to deliver a brief therapy (see chapter ten, by Alessandra Lemma, Mary Target, & Peter Fonagy), or to meet the needs of patients with antisocial personality disorder (chapter eight, by Jessica Yakeley), or to inform the development of online therapeutic interventions (chapter nine, by Richard Graham), or to complement the work of allied physical and mental health professionals (chapter five, by Rock & Carrington) is sometimes unhelpfully conflated with a dilution of psychoanalysis and, as such, is regarded as not *really* psychoanalytic—a bastard offspring of the so-called real thing.

To keep alive the invaluable contribution that psychoanalysis can make to Public Mental Health, and for it to take up its legitimate place within a modern health-care economy, it is vital that it adapts and evolves to meet the various diverse needs of patients (Lemma & Patrick, 2010). This process does not dilute the "real thing"—rather, it modifies an earlier model: this is development, which inevitably comes with loss. Not engaging in this process of adaptation and change only serves to marginalize psychoanalysis further in what has undeniably become an inhospitable external climate in this respect. Change is always destabilizing, but relinquishing the old need not entail compromising core values or defacing the valuable contributions made by other colleagues at different points in time. This thing that we call "new" can never be new in any absolute sense: it always has a history that informs it and out of which it has grown. It is very much in this spirit that these four chapters need to be read.

All of the contributors in Part III speak to the value of integrating different ways of working and the importance of collaboration with other organizations/services in order to meet the challenge of complexity. The fluency with which they describe these developments conceals the hard work that makes such integration possible within a team and across organizations. Any institution wishing to provide integrated, multimodel services will require organizational structures that can contain and manage group processes so as to create spaces that allow for difference to be an asset rather than a threat.

When pluralism can be tolerated and the anxieties it promotes can be constructively managed, we have much to gain, as the work of the clinicians in this book testifies. Ultimately, it does not matter if everyone's final vocabulary is different. Sameness is not what we should be aspiring to, but there should be enough overlap to allow for everybody to realize the desirability of engaging with other belief systems as well as one's own.

References

Lemma, A., & Johnston, J. (2010). Editorial. *Psychoanalytic Psychotherapy*, 24 (3): 179–182.

Lemma, A., & Patrick, M. (2010). Contemporary psychoanalytic applications: Development and its vicissitudes. In: A. Lemma & M. Patrick (Eds.), *Off the Couch: Contemporary Psychoanalytic Applications*. London: Routledge.

CHAPTER EIGHT

Treating the untreatable: the evolution of a psychoanalytically informed service for antisocial personality disorder

Jessica Yakeley

People tend to define and categorize themselves and others on the basis of appearance and behaviours. While attitudes towards certain types of appearance (such as skin colour) or behaviours (such as homosexual acts) have become more tolerant, other sexual and aggressive behaviours have become less acceptable to today's society, which is more likely to react with punitive and ostracizing measures in the name of public protection than attempt to analyse the complex underlying dynamics and motivations of the person involved. It is as if the individuals behind the behaviours have been lost from view, and, more specifically, their minds and the complex contents and processes within are forgotten or dismissed as simply bad.

The field of mental health has not escaped the myopic tendency to focus on the most obvious behavioural manifestations of human activities at the expense of the much more uncertain endeavour of exploring the mind. Mental illnesses and disorders of personality are diagnostically categorized on the basis of observable symptoms, signs, and behaviours, regardless of aetiological theories. Antisocial personality disorder (ASPD) is a syndrome affecting approximately 1% of the male population (Coid, Yang, Tyrer, Roberts, & Ullrich, 2006;

Torgensen, Kringlen, & Cramer, 2001) that is defined largely by behavioural criteria, particularly those emphasizing criminality. This is one reason why many people with a diagnosis of ASPD have contact with the criminal justice system, where their behaviours are punished, but may have little or no contact with the mental health system, as they are thought undeserving or unsuitable for treatment. Their plight has been exacerbated by the constant reorganization of community and forensic psychiatric services, with a primary focus on treating mental illness rather than personality disorder. Such fragmentation of service provision mirrors the disrupted lives and chaotic inner worlds of these difficult patients, and those who do seek treatment often find themselves being referred from service to service—a repetition of their early attachment history.

This chapter explores how certain individuals who are categorized on the basis of and alienated by their antisocial behaviour may be thought about in relation to their minds and examines how they may benefit from a psychological treatment approach, mentalization (Bateman & Fonagy, 2004), which focuses explicitly on minds in relation to other minds. I describe the thinking behind an evolving service at the Portman Clinic for the treatment of patients with a diagnosis of ASPD. Such patients have traditionally been thought to be untreatable with psychoanalytic psychotherapy. This pessimism is due to the difficulties of engaging with patients whose deception and emotional detachment may foreclose any possibility of entering into a viable therapeutic relationship and where the focus of therapy is constantly being diverted from exploration of the patient's mind into managing their risky antisocial behaviours.

Although there is a lack of systematic controlled empirical evidence indicating that psychodynamic treatments are effective in this group of individuals, more recent research, suggesting that ASPD is a disorder of attachment (Frodi, Dernevik, Sepa, Philipson, & Bragesio, 2001; Levinson & Fonagy, 2004; van IJzendoorn et al., 1997), is stimulating a renewed interest in psychodynamic approaches. This parallels the move towards taking a more dimensional approach in the diagnosis of personality disorder, reflecting a consideration of underlying structural dynamics rather than just surface symptomatology. This conceptual understanding of ASPD as a disorder of attachment with both biological and psychological determinants has led us to modify and refine our therapeutic technique and treatment model for these patients. Specifically, we are developing a mentalization-based treatment intervention for men with a diagnosis of ASPD, embedded in a psychoanalytically informed setting with a particular model of containment and management of risk. In this chapter, I describe the theoretical underpinnings of this model of intervention, as well as some of the difficulties and challenges encountered in setting up the project, which tested the boundaries of our own interpersonal behaviour and professional relationships.

Diagnostic controversy and confusion

What is antisocial personality disorder? According to the American Psychiatric Association's *Diagnostic and Statistical Manual of Mental Disorders* (DSM–IV; APA, 1994), personality disorders are defined as variations or exaggerations of normal personality attributes and traits that cannot be diagnosed before the age of 18 years and involve "enduring patterns of cognition, affectivity, interpersonal behaviour and impulse control that are culturally deviant, pervasive and inflexible, leading to distress and social impairment, and in some cases antisocial behaviour". Antisocial behaviours constitute, not surprisingly, the main diagnostic features of ASPD, and such individuals must show, according to DSM–IV, some or all of the following abnormal behaviours and personality traits: a pervasive pattern of disregard for and violation of rights of others, a failure to conform to social norms, deceitfulness, impulsivity or failure to plan ahead, irritability and aggressiveness, reckless disregard for safety of self and others, consistent irresponsibility, and lack of remorse. The World Health Organization's *International Statistical Classification of Diseases and Related Health Problems* (ICD-10; WHO, 1992) provides a similar descriptive list of behavioural items that constitute "dissocial personality disorder", the equivalent of DSM–IV's antisocial personality disorder.

However, these contemporary psychiatric diagnostic classification systems, which are based on descriptive phenomenology and use a categorical approach to classify disorders on the basis of observable behaviours and symptoms rather than theories of causation, become problematic when applied to the diagnosis of personality disorder. This is particularly relevant for the current diagnoses of antisocial or dissocial personality disorder, which describe constellations of behaviours that may in fact be the outcome of different aetiological pathways. There is increasing evidence that both biological and environmental factors can interact in complex ways and to varying degrees to produce different forms of the disorder. Although numerous studies have shown that genetic, neuro-anatomical, and biochemical factors are implicated in ASPD (e.g. Viding, Larsson, & Jones, 2008), research also shows that the incidence of childhood neglect, abuse, trauma, and loss is much higher in people with ASPD than in the normal population. This is in accord with the clinical experience of working with people with personality disorder, who often report histories of disrupted childhoods during which they were not only abused and neglected, but may also have experienced parental mental illness and alcoholism, poverty, unemployment, domestic violence, family breakdown, and periods of time in care.

Research into the causes of ASPD has been hampered by lack of clarity regarding the definition of the disorder. The term "psychopathy" is often used interchangeably with ASPD. However, it is more useful to conceptualize and assess psychopathy as one of the personality dimensions or traits, exhibited in callousness and lack of remorse, that make up the antisocial syndrome, which can differ in severity in different forms of the disorder. This approach is more useful when considering treatment and reflects the thrust of personality research in general towards dimensional rather than categorical measures (Livesley, 2004; Patrick, 2006). A dimensional approach assumes quantitative differences, or varying degrees of dysfunction, and shifts the focus of personality disorder from surface psychopathology to a consideration of underlying structural abnormalities and deficits in character, which is more compatible with psychoanalytic conceptualizations. Indeed, it is likely that a dimensional approach will feature more prominently in the next version of the American diagnostic manual, DSM–V. There is ample evidence to suggest that higher psychopathy scores predict a poorer response to treatment (Hare, 1991) and reflect a more severe form of personality disorder that is likely to have a considerable genetic and biological basis. However, we can identify another substantial group of individuals under the ASPD umbrella, whose psychopathology may be more determined by early environmental adversity that exerts its pathogenicity on the early psychological development of the person, specifically via disruption to the attachment process.

A disorder of attachment and mentalization

Following Bowlby, researchers into the study of attachment have shown that the early relationship to the primary caregivers is critical to the development of personality, mental representations, and affect control. Fonagy and colleagues (Bateman & Fonagy, 2004; Fonagy, Moran, & Target, 1993; Fonagy, Steele, Steele, Moran, & Higgitt, 1991; Fonagy & Target, 1995) have extended the field of attachment research by introducing the concept of mentalization, which they propose is a fundamental process underpinning the normal development of mind. Mentalization is the capacity to reflect and to think about one's mental states, including thoughts, beliefs, desires, and affects, to be able to distinguish one's own mental states from others, and to be able to interpret the actions of oneself and others as meaningful and based on intentional mental states. The normal development of mentalization is dependent on the intersubjective process of emerging psychological awareness between the child and his primary caregivers in the context of a secure attachment. The child becomes increasingly aware of his own mind through his growing awareness of the mind of his mother via her capacity to demonstrate to him that she thinks of him as a separate person, with his own distinct intentions, beliefs, and desires. The mother who is not attuned to her baby's experience will provide inadequate mirroring of the infant's behaviour (Winnicott, 1956), so that the child is unable to develop a representation of his own experience and, instead, internalizes the image of the caregiver. Where the mother or primary caregiver has been neglectful or frankly malevolent towards the child, as in the case of many individuals with ASPD, this internalized representation will be experienced as foreign or bad and will never be fully integrated into his overall schema of self-representations. Bateman and Fonagy (2008) have called this discontinuity within the self the "alien self" and suggest that this internalized self-representation is continually subject to the pressure of projection into others to maintain the illusion of a self that does not contain unacceptable aspects.

For people with ASPD, this pattern of relating persists into adulthood. They are dependent on relationships with others into whom they can project alien aspects of themselves in order to stabilize their minds and feel a sense of self-coherence. Relationships in individuals with ASPD tend to be rigid, hierarchical, and controlling, as exemplified in dismissive attitudes towards women, who are viewed as inferior, or in the "gang culture" of organized crime. Notions of recognition and respect assume a special importance in their interpersonal relationships. When such relationships are challenged by the other person refusing to be the recipient of malign projections, as in the previously subjugated wife who now talks back to her abusive husband, the return of the alien self threatens the person's fragile stability of mind, leading to unbearable feelings of shame and humiliation (Gilligan, 1996), which may lead to violence in an attempt to regain control and sense of integrity.

Fonagy and Target (1996, 2000, 2007; Target & Fonagy, 1996) have identified several primitive or pre-mentalistic modes of thinking that predate the emergence of mentalization. These are present in the normal early childhood development of all of us but persist and predominate in people with certain personality disorders. These pre-mentalistic modes of organizing subjective experience include psychic equivalence, pretend mode, and teleological thinking. Psychic equivalence is often referred to as concrete thinking, where internal and external reality are experienced as isomorphic, there is no tolerance of differing points of view, and thoughts cannot be symbolized. In pretend mode, thoughts and feelings are dissociated from reality to the point of meaninglessness, so that a person may appear to be talking about important internal experiences, but these are disconnected from any meaningful context. Teleological mode refers a mode of thinking in which the motivations of others are interpreted according to the presence of physical actions. Here, changes in mental states are only felt to be real when confirmed by physically observable action—for example, the person who only believes that her boyfriend cares about her if he buys her flowers; if he does not, this is proof that he does not care.

Bateman and Fonagy (2008) suggest that the descriptive phenomena of ASPD are due to a regression from mentalistic ways of viewing the world to pre-mentalistic modes. The person with ASPD experiences psychic stability so long as projection of the alien self remains successful, but when this fails, pre-mentalistic types of thinking emerge, especially teleological thinking. They propose that reactive violence in individuals with ASPD is triggered by these inhibitions or failures in the capacity for mentalization. In reactive violence, sometimes called affective violence (Meloy, 1992) or self-preservative violence (Glasser, 1998), the person is highly sensitive to threats to his or her self-worth or "respect", causing internal emotional states of shame and humiliation, which are experienced as threatening his or her very psychic survival. This triggers a collapse in mental functioning as such unbearable feelings cannot be managed by representational means within the mind but are now experienced very concretely in psychic equivalence mode as feelings that the person needs to expel in violent action. The loss of mentalization also means that the person is unable to empathize with his or her victim or consider different motivations in the victim's mind, which would normally inhibit violence towards others, and, moreover, the onset of pretend mode creates an illusory sense of safety in which the violent person is detached from reality and hence the danger and consequences of his or her actions. Violence here is therefore defensive, as opposed to the more cold, calculating, and planned psychopathic (Meloy, 1992) or sadistic (Glasser, 1998) violence seen in psychopathic individuals.

Bateman and Fonagy (2011) propose that a substantial group of patients who fulfil current diagnostic criteria for ASPD have experienced significant trauma and disruptions to their attachment system in childhood, which has interfered with their neurobiological development and the development of psychological defences, compromising their mentalization capacity and lowering their threshold for emotional reactivity. It is important to consider that the callous and unemotional behaviour of some children assumed to have constitutional abnormalities (Barry et al, 2000; Lynam & Gudonis, 2005) may also be rooted in attachment difficulties, and that such behaviour may not be a primary abnormality but a defence against anxiety. Empirical evidence to support the hypothesis that ASPD is a developmental disorder rooted in attachment comes from studies showing abnormal attachment patterns in forensic patients and prisoners diagnosed with ASPD (Frodi et al., 2001; Levinson & Fonagy, 2004; van IJzendoorn et al., 1997).

Where is the violence?

In recent years the demography of the Portman Clinic's patient population has significantly altered. Although the Clinic's first formal patient, seen in 1933, was a violent woman—"a woman, 47 years of age, noted as having a violent temper, charged with assault on her woman employer" (Saville & Rumney, 1992)—the majority of patients referred to the Clinic today are male. Moreover, the proportion of violent to perverse patients has diminished, with fewer referrals of cases of violent behaviour, in contrast to those of perverse sexual behaviour, who now make up the majority of the patients referred and accepted for assessment and treatment. The reasons for this are speculative and complex. Society is currently preoccupied with an apparent endemic of paedophilia, largely exposed by the Internet with the discovery and arrest of thousands of individuals caught accessing Internet child pornography, many of whom presumably would previously never have reached the attention of the authorities. In the last few years the Portman Clinic has correspondingly received many more referrals of people addicted to adult and child pornography, many of whom are middle class and educated and perhaps therefore more able to access treatment.

Although aggression is inherent in these paraphilic conditions, fewer cases of overt violence with no obvious sexual component are being referred for psychotherapeutic treatment. There is no evidence that violence and antisocial behaviour in society has decreased: if anything, it has remained stable or increased in certain populations (Home Office, 2006; Ministry of Justice, 2008). However, violent individuals who enter the criminal justice system may be less likely to be referred for outpatient treatment than before, as the prevailing emphasis on public protection means that the management of offenders prioritizes punishment and restraint over therapeutics. Moreover, fewer probation officers than before are familiar with a psychodynamic therapeutic model, as most treatment programmes for offenders, such as anger management, are based on a cognitive behavioural model focusing on abnormal behaviour rather than underlying characterological and interpersonal difficulties. Another factor is that psychiatrists have traditionally held an ambivalent attitude towards the relationship between violence and mental disorder. A patient whose violence is clearly associated with a mental illness, generally schizophrenia, will be accepted for treatment, usually in a secure institution, where he or she will be treated with antipsychotic medication. However, although violence may be equated with madness in the public imagination, psychotic violence is in fact rare, accounting for only a small proportion of all serious incidents of violence (Tardiff, 2003). Long-standing personality traits such as impulsivity, aggression, and interpersonal deficits are more likely to be associated with violent behaviour.

However, many psychiatrists and mental health services have refused to treat individuals with a primary diagnosis of personality disorder. This may be because they do not believe they have the skills or resources to treat these patients, but it may also be explained by an unacknowledged countertransferential response that unconsciously defends against the powerful and uncomfortable feelings evoked by personality-disordered patients, many of whom do not willingly accept treatment and lead clinicians to feel angry, despondent, or doubting their own professional capacities. One might speculate that the tenacity of the misconception that personality disorder is untreatable and intractable arises from a rationalization of clinicians' unwillingness to have contact with such patients, rather than a belief based on objective evidence. Personality-disordered patients have historically been treated at the margins of the health service, often presenting to accident and emergency services or primary care where they are treated for acute medical or psychiatric crises but where their personality difficulties are missed. An inconsistent approach by secondary psychiatric services has resulted in such individuals being either denied assessment altogether or inappropriately admitted to inpatient general psychiatric wards, as many community teams and outpatient services feel ill-equipped to cope with the demands of these patients.

The lack of suitable services for individuals with a diagnosis of personality disorder was highlighted in a key government document published in 2003, *Personality Disorder—No Longer a Diagnosis of Exclusion* (DoH, 2003). This led to a significant expansion in the development and provision of specialized services in the United Kingdom for personality-disordered patients, particularly those with a diagnosis of borderline or emotionally unstable personality disorder. However, people with a diagnosis of ASPD remain on the periphery of mental health, and access for such individuals to suitable treatment is limited. It is perhaps difficult to see the psychological disturbance in people who display violent and antisocial behaviour towards others, where their mental anguish is disowned and projected so that those around them suffer. Such individuals are more likely to evoke a punitive than therapeutic response and are routed through the criminal justice system, where their psychological difficulties are missed. Health care facilities in prisons are often inadequate, and psychiatric treatment is limited to prisoners who show signs of clear-cut mental illness rather than personality disorder (DoH, 2009). Within forensic services, many regional secure units continue to actively exclude patients with a primary diagnosis of personality disorder and will accept patients only if they have a co-morbid diagnosis of a mental illness—usually schizophrenia. Forensic psychiatric and psychology outpatient services also vary significantly in their referral criteria, with many offering limited if any services for personality disorder. For a small number of individuals designated as suffering from "dangerous and severe personality disorder" (DSPD), a limited number of services have been set up in the last decade, piloted and researched by the Department of Health (DoH, 1999). These individuals are judged to be suffering from a serious disorder of personality, which accounts for their high risk to others. However, most people who might fulfil diagnostic criteria for ASPD are not judged dangerous enough to be suitable for these DSPD services.

We have therefore identified a considerable service gap in the mental health market for patients with a diagnosis of ASPD, particularly in the provision of outpatient psychological treatments. Could the Portman Clinic, with its previous rich experience and expertise in the psychoanalytic understanding and treatment of people who are violent, contribute to the development of services for patients with a disorder of personality previously thought to be untreatable, and where the current aetiological research emphasis is biogenetic? And would this constructively re-address the current imbalance in referrals to the Portman Clinic by reclaiming the treatment ground for patients who are violent, or would this create unmanageable anxieties and unnecessary risks for both patients and staff? Before specifically addressing these questions, it is worth reviewing the research evidence to date regarding the treatment studies of this disorder and the diagnostic and conceptual foundations on which such studies are based.

An untreatable disorder

The early literature on individual psychoanalytic therapy (Cleckley, 1941; Freud, 1916d) and group psychotherapy (Foulkes, 1948) for antisocial patients was based on individual case reports, and it is likely that the most disturbed individuals were not offered treatment (McGauley, Adshead, & Sarkar, 2007). Because of the high levels of dangerous acting-out behaviours on the part of patients with ASPD, such as violence, self-harm, substance abuse, and infraction of the law, attempts to treat these patients with conventional outpatient psychotherapy have rarely been successful (Gabbard & Coyne, 1987; Meloy, 1995). It was recognized that such patients needed to be seen in an institutional setting to provide sufficient containment of the risks that they posed for any effective therapeutic intervention to take place safely. However, admission to a general psychiatric hospital has not been shown to be helpful for most antisocial patients, as these patients tend to disrupt the ward by rule-breaking, smuggling in alcohol and drugs, assaulting patients and staff, or by more subtle corruption such as undermining other patients' therapeutic alliances with staff, or seducing professionals into unethical behaviour (Gabbard, 2005). The more psychopathic the patient, the more likely it is that he or she will convert what is meant to be a therapeutic experience into an exploitative one to gratify his or her pathological and perverse needs, leaving staff feeling deceived, humiliated, and demoralized.

This led to the development of specialized institutional settings for the treatment of antisocial and psychopathic patients and offenders, in both the mental health and criminal justice systems. Here, the environmental setting, or milieu, can become an essential therapeutic tool of the therapy, in which behaviour can be challenged and modified. The therapeutic community is a long-standing model of treatment that developed from the interest in group treatments after the Second World War (Jones, 1952), but it has only recently been subjected to empirical evaluation. In the United Kingdom, most of the research on the efficacy of therapeutic community treatment has been on the work of the Henderson Hospital, a residential therapeutic community funded for many years by the National Health Service. Therapeutic communities have also been developed in prisons: in the United Kingdom, the best-known of these is HMP Grendon Underwood, a specialist prison for males with personality disorder. A review of treatments for ASPD and psychopathic disorder (Dolan & Coid, 1993) suggested that therapeutic community approaches showed the most promising forms of treatment for psychopathic disorder, but the authors also noted the lack of scientific rigor for all of the treatment studies reviewed.

McGauley, Adshead, and Sarkar (2007) highlight how this cautious optimism was seriously dented by a series of studies in the 1990s showing that group interventions in therapeutic community settings for psychopaths not only had a poorer treatment response and greater dropout rate than those for non-psychopaths (Ogloff, Wong, & Greenwood, 1990), but actually increased violent recidivism in the psychopathic population studied (Harris, Rice, & Cormier, 1991, 1994). This led to a widespread belief that psychopathic and ASPD patients were untreatable, which influenced the development of treatment services as well as mental health legislation. Subsequent research has, however, challenged the view that psychopathy is untreatable. Recent meta-analyses of the effectiveness of psychological therapies in treating personality disorder, including psychopathy (D'Silva, Duggan, & McCarthy, 2004; Duggan et al., 2006; Salekin, 2002), suggest that such disorders may indeed be treatable, although further randomized controlled trials are necessary. Overall, it was found that lengthier and more intensive treatments were significantly more effective.

In the past two decades, following a series of high-profile homicides widely reported by the media, much of the interest in the treatment of ASPD has been fuelled by increasing political concern about public protection from mentally ill offenders. This led to the setting up, in the United Kingdom, of specialized intensive units for patients with severe personality disorders—so-called dangerous and severe personality disorder (DSPD) individuals—who present significant risk of harm to others, linked to their personality disorder (DoH and Home Office, 1999). Although many mental health and civil liberties activists objected to the fact that DSPD is not a clinical diagnosis and could potentially lead to individuals being locked up *before* they had committed an offence, many also acknowledged the lack of comprehensive service provision that exists world-wide—with the possible exception of the Netherlands—for the treatment of high-risk personality-disordered offenders. Pilot forensic personality disorder services were set up within both high and medium secure psychiatric hospitals and in prisons, as well as in the community. However, although full evaluation of these units and their treatment will not be completed for some years, the DSPD programme is being disbanded, largely due to its poor cost-effectiveness.

In recent years, cognitive behavioural therapies targeting the antisocial personality-disordered patient's problematic behaviours and associated symptoms, such as aggression, self-harm, and substance abuse, have been promoted over therapies aimed at altering the underlying core abnormal personality structure. However, the research methodology involved in evaluating these various treatments remains problematic, with confusion over diagnostic criteria and conceptualizations of psychopathy, differences in defining and measuring outcome, and a focus on behavioural and symptomatic rather than structural personality change. The recently issued NICE guidelines on ASPD (NICE, 2009) are to be welcomed in drawing attention to ASPD. However, the guidelines focus on early intervention strategies aimed at the parents and families of children at risk of developing conduct disorder who may go on to develop ASPD, whereas the treatment approaches recommended for adults with the disorder are limited. These guidelines highlight the need to re-examine some of the nosological and aetiological assumptions that underpin the treatment rationale of this disorder and lead us beyond the impasse of the nurture-versus-nature dichotomy.

Mentalization-based treatment
for antisocial personality disorder

Mentalization-based treatment (MBT) is a therapeutic approach based on the above theoretical principles of mentalization, originally developed for the treatment of patients with borderline personality disorder (BPD) (Bateman & Fonagy, 2004, 2006). This is a relational approach, where the person's mind and his or her relationship with other minds are the foci of therapy. MBT differs from cognitive behavioural therapy in attempting to treat other aspects of personality dysfunction rather than just focusing on behaviours.

The project being described in this chapter is an attempt to adapt this treatment model to patients with a diagnosis of ASPD. As we saw earlier, people with ASPD—like patients with BPD—revert to pre-mentalistic modes of thinking when their attachment relationships are threatened, and identifying such experiences and consequent shifts in thinking is a prime focus of the treatment. However, in people with ASPD, mentalization—in particular, the externalization of the alien self—is quite rigid, and challenging their fragile state of psychic equilibrium by asking them to consider and re-own projected parts of themselves they consider unacceptable risks provoking a violent response. Therapeutic interventions must therefore be carefully formulated and delivered in a manner that does not cause patients to feel overwhelmed by unbearable affect to the point that they mount an aggressive defence that could put others and themselves at risk.

I do not here provide a comprehensive description of the technique of MBT, which the reader can find elsewhere (Bateman & Fonagy, 2004, 2006), but highlight some of the technical challenges and dilemmas that we are encountering in our attempt to treat this particular patient group. One of the overall aims of treatment is to facilitate such patients in their interpersonal functioning by stimulating attachment bonds while encouraging them to examine the mental states they experience in relation to others. This process may be more effective in group treatment, as this offers more opportunities to understand other people's minds and is less arousing than individual therapy. This is important for many patients with ASPD who may be quite paranoid, and their tendency to perceive the world in psychic equivalence mode means that in individual work they may form erotic or even psychotic transference relationships with the therapist. In a group setting, the multiple transferences available dilute the intensity of feeling and offer patients more than one target for their aggression, which may be reassuring. In our experience, the patients are initially wary of being critical of each other, and the therapists must tolerate being the targets of their aggression and resentments for a long time, until the patients feel safe enough to challenge each other's points of view.

The current treatment framework involves the patient participating in a weekly MBT group run by two therapists, and a monthly individual session with one of the group therapists. In the latter, the clinician continues to adopt a mentalizing approach and uses the individual meeting to support the patient's ongoing participation in the group by allowing him or her the opportunity to discuss any difficulties he or she might be experiencing in the group. Although many patients may express anxieties about participating in group treatment and have a preference for the individual attention afforded in the one-to-one setting, it is made clear to the patient that the group is the main modality of treatment, and an individual session will only be offered once the patient has attended at least three consecutive group meetings.

The majority of patients with ASPD do not accept that they have mental health difficulties, and many will reject treatment. Although all of the patients in our group have presented voluntarily to mental health services seeking treatment for anger, depression, and anxiety, the experience of being a psychotherapy patient can be deeply humiliating, and, not surprisingly, we have found them difficult to engage in ongoing treatment following the initial assessment. This has necessitated a more assertive approach on our part than is conventional in psychodynamic therapy, such as telephone contact with the patient after missed sessions, encouraging him to attend, and adopting a more psychoeducational approach in initial sessions to explain the treatment model. However, to discourage those patients who seek treatment solely to be seen in a better light by external authorities such as the courts, probation, or housing, it is made clear to them that we will not provide reports on their treatment progress to these external bodies in the first few months of treatment, until some genuine motivation for change is evident in the patient.

This brings us to rules and boundaries, which are important in any group treatment but can become a central feature in groups for ASPD. Many individuals with ASPD will have a distrust of parental figures and institutions of authority, often based on their earlier experiences of being unfairly treated. At the same time, they often belong to groups, such as gangs or organized criminal syndicates, which, while in opposition to societal authority, have their own internal hierarchical structures, code of honour, and leaders. Developing a sense of responsibility and awareness of appropriate boundaries in relation to others is an essential task of treatment. The antisocial person will inevitably react against whatever rules he or she feels are imposed upon him or her, and the group therapists must permit the expression of anti-authoritarian attitudes without these becoming destructive to the group. The group therapists must set the group rules in order for the group to feel safe, but they must be prepared to represent parental authority figures against whom the group can rebel. A critical role for the therapists is to carry the patient's alien self, which can only be explored once the patient feels safe and contained. ASPD patients experience the world in terms of power and control, and this paradigm will inevitably colour their relationship with the therapists. However, early interpretations of the transference should be avoided, as this can stimulate feelings of humiliation; the therapist should, instead, readily apologize for perceived errors and accept criticism to counteract the patient's expectations that the therapists hold all the power.

The therapist's stance is important in modelling a mentalizing attitude and establishing an appropriate shared code of conduct in the group. The therapist aims to promote an atmosphere of concerned inquiry about what is happening in patients' minds, rather than condemnation or an "all-knowing" attitude. This involves taking a non-judgmental stance and speaking to the patients in an authentic, direct, and respectful manner, while avoiding opaqueness, hesitancy, and secrecy. The aim is to nurture trust, openness, and honesty in the context of attachment relationships with the other group members, by first highlighting and exploring their own code of conduct and interactions with others within and outside the group. Group discussions are focused on the patients' violent and aggressive behaviours, and patients are encouraged to think about the events that led up to the violent event and the thoughts and feelings they were experiencing at the time. We have found that without active intervention, group members tend to drift into wider pseudo-philosophical discussions about the problems of society where people will always take advantage of others. While this may represent an attempt to form a common bond in a paranoid view of the world, this also marks a shift into pretend mode, and the aim is to bring them back to focusing on recent specific behaviours and to link these to their internal mental states.

A further difficulty is presented in attempting to foster an interest in each other on the part of group members. Patients with ASPD, particularly the more psychopathic ones, may appear to show some enhanced areas of mentalization in their ability to deceive and exploit others, which necessitates an ability to understand the mind of the other. This is, however, mind-reading without empathizing (Baron-Cohen, 2005), and this apparently highly tuned capacity to mentalize is actually restricted and is rarely generalizable to complex interpersonal situations (Bateman & Fonagy, 2006). In our group we have observed a lack of empathic interest in each others' mental processes when relaying their accounts of incidents, and it has been difficult to get group members to question each other. The first step, therefore, has been to encourage the patients to focus on their own internal states and how they are made to feel by others rather than asking them to consider how another person feels. However, the patients' anger can be easily activated when describing emotive topics, at which point their mentalization ceases, and the therapists need to actively intervene in the form of a "stop rewind". Here, attention is deflected away from the angry member until his or her state of arousal diminishes by encouraging the other group members to examine what has just occurred in the group to make that person angry, or for therapists themselves to offer their opinions if the patients are unable to reflect on the situation.

Managing risks and tensions

The most obvious risk to be managed in offering a service to patients with ASPD is that of violence. Before they are offered treatment, all of the patients will have been carefully assessed over several meetings with one of the group therapists, both of whom are Consultant Psychiatrists in Forensic Psychotherapy, which will include formal assessment of their risk of violence using the HCR-20 (Historical Clinical Risk-20; Webster, Douglas, Eaves, & Hart, 1997), which includes a measure of psychopathy with the PCL–R (Psychopathy Checklist–Revised; Hare, 2003). Patients with high psychopathy scores (over 30) are excluded from the project, as are patients with a diagnosis of psychosis and those who are dependent on alcohol or drugs. At the assessment stage it is important that the therapists liaise actively with the patient's GP and other mental health services involved with the patient, particularly the patient's CMHT or forensic psychiatric service, if necessary. This is not only to gain a forensic psychiatric opinion of the patient but to establish where the patient may be referred to in an emergency if his mental state breaks down, given that the Portman Clinic is not an inpatient facility. The risk of self-harm and suicide may be overlooked when the focus has historically been on the patient's violence in relation to others, but suicidal impulses may become more prominent in treatment as the patient becomes aware of mental states that he has previously defended against. Many of the patients will already have had a general or forensic psychiatric assessment but then not thought suitable for the respective service, and we have found it necessary to be assertive at times with colleagues in other services about the need for their continued involvement, even if the patient is seen infrequently by the external service. Such external support is critical not only for the overall containment of the patient and the risks that he poses, but also to manage the anxieties of the therapists working directly with these patients.

It may also be necessary to establish contact with other agencies involved with the patient, such as the probation service and, in some cases, Multi-agency Public Protection Arrangements (MAPPA), but this should at all times be discussed openly with the patient, and the lines of communication and boundaries regarding information sharing and confidentiality should be transparent. Managing the tension between confidentiality and disclosure is at the heart of work with forensic patients. The recent preoccupation with risk assessment and

management of offenders has encouraged the sharing of information between professionals and agencies, but this is at odds with the
patient's right to confidentiality in the therapeutic setting, and they
may not engage in treatment if their confidentiality is compromised.
We have found that ASPD patients appear reassured by our policy of
not reporting the content of sessions to external agencies unless we
consider there to be a current and serious risk of harm to themselves
or others. This allows them to feel freer in discussing their violent fantasies and actions in the group without the risk of routine disclosure,
but to feel contained by knowing that we will impose a boundary
if necessary. This is consistent with a mentalizing stance in which
the therapist does not condone or collude with the patient's violent
state of mind—this would be psychic equivalence—but can offer a
different point of view, which may occasionally necessitate acting by
informing others of the patient's risk. Such actions may, of course,
be experienced by the patient in teleological mode, but this may be
explored with the patient as part of the therapeutic work.

Integrating the new with the old

In our experience to date of running the group for ASPD patients,
although they report incidents of minor violence in their external lives
between sessions, which form an important focus of the group discussions, we have had only one violent incident in the group session, in
which a patient became angry and kicked a table. Although this was
taken very seriously by the group at the time, and the other patients
were subsequently able to usefully mentalize the angry patient's feelings that led to his outburst, there have been no further aggressive
incidents in the clinic. It appears that the patients are more likely to
not attend the group rather than become violent within the treatment setting. This observation has, however, not allayed the fears
of other clinicians and staff working in the clinic in relation to this
new service. Although the Portman Clinic has always treated violent
patients, these have never been formally categorized or diagnosed as
having ASPD, although presumably many former violent patients of
the clinic would have fulfilled the diagnostic criteria. There seemed
to be a belief that we were embarking on accepting a much more
disturbed, and hence dangerous, group of patients than had previ-

ously been treated at the Clinic. Anxieties and fantasies seemed to proliferate, not just among the clinicians, but also the administrative staff, creating an atmosphere of tension but also concealed excitement in the period of assessment of patients leading up to the start of the group. This culminated in an incident of violence from a patient who was not in the group for ASPD patients, which had not yet started, but in one of the long-standing mixed groups for patients suffering from perversions as well as violence. It was as if the anxieties about starting this new service could not be contained and had spilled over into the Clinic as a whole.

There was also openly expressed concern and criticism about departing from practising conventional psychoanalytic psychother-apy and delivering a new treatment model, which was perceived by a significant minority of therapists at the Portman and in the wider Trust to be antithetical to psychoanalysis, and which, moreover, they feared, would exacerbate the patients' anxieties and increase the risk of violent enactment. Such critical responses became more overt concerning our decision to video record the group sessions for super-vision and research purposes. Such an intervention was considered to be a major intrusion in the therapeutic setting, which would increase the patients' levels of paranoia and hence elevate their risk. In fact, most of the patients appear to quickly accept the presence of the camera, and any questions and fears about it are openly discussed.

It appeared that some of the staff's criticisms were based more on fear of change rather than on a full understanding and informed critique of the MBT treatment model. The introduction of an explic-itly modified therapy model also exposed pre-existing differences in psychotherapeutic theory and technique among the clinical staff. In order to address this constructively, we organized meetings for the whole clinic staff in which the project could be candidly presented and debated.

Although there are obvious differences in technique between psy-choanalytic psychotherapy and MBT, there are also many points of convergence. Fonagy and Bateman (2010) describe the history of MBT and its roots in psychoanalytic theory and practice, and how the model has been influenced by the writings of psychoanalysts working with borderline and narcissistic pathology such as Bion, Glasser, Green, Kernberg, Mahler, Racker, Rosenfeld, and Winnicott, as well as developmental work with children carried out at the Anna Freud Centre. It should also be emphasized that MBT was developed specifically for patients with BPD, and our project aims to adapt the model for another specific group of patients, those with ASPD, whose psychopathology is similarly based in a disorder of attachment and who are widely thought not to be suitable for psychoanalytic psycho-therapy. The reluctance that some psychoanalytic therapists may have in viewing MBT as emerging from the stable of applied psychoana-lytic therapies may also reflect the ambiguous place of attachment in psychoanalytic theory. Although MBT is not the treatment of choice for all patients, it can be usefully added to the array of treatments offered to a very specific patient population, namely ASPD.

Focusing too much on the specific treatment model neglects think-ing about the wider institution and the layers of containment that this offers. I would suggest that Portman MBT could be seen as a newer model embedded within an older and wider one. This is a psycho-analytic model of containment, which has within it reflective spaces at many levels where the patients' violent actions, and their underlying affects, defences, and fantasies, may be thought about and processed. This is both an intrapsychic and an interpersonal process, influenced by Bion's concept of containment in relation to maternal reverie in the mother–infant relationship (Bion, 1959, 1962) and Winnicott's related notion of maternal holding (Winnicott, 1954), where the presence of others who can provide therapeutic relationships is paramount.

In the first instance, the group therapists, by their mentaliz-ing functions, provide an intermediary space where actions can be thought about and thoughts can be played with. At the same time they act as containers of the patients' unmanageable affects, embod-ied in the alien self, until these can be processed and fed back to the patient in a more manageable form. However, containment is not sufficient without triangulation—that is, the presence of a third per-spective, from minds that are more removed from the immediacy of the therapeutic encounter and can hence offer a more "objective" viewpoint. Although group treatment offers several minds in its different members who may offer different viewpoints, powerful unconscious group processes and defences, which Bion called "basic assumption groups" (Bion, 1961), may operate and undermine the more conscious and manifest work of the group, and so the input of an independent supervisor can be helpful. We have therefore arranged for regular supervision with one of the founders of MBT, with whom we view and discuss the videotapes of the group ses-sions. The patients themselves have access to an independent psychiatrist within the clinic, who acts as "case manager" and will, occasionally, see the patients for matters that do not appear to able to be resolved within the group.

The ASPD service is also supported by the many different reflective forums that exist to support all of the therapeutic work at the Portman Clinic. These reflective meetings aid the therapists in processing their often disturbing countertransferences to the patients. They can be thought of as providing a paternal function in conjunction with the maternal aspects of the therapist, to create a more healthy parental couple that can think constructively about the patients—an experience that most have never had (Britton, 1989).

Finally, the tensions that emerged around the inception of this new service may be symptoms reflecting the uneasy position of forensic psychotherapy in the wider world. Forensic psychotherapy in the NHS falls at the intersection of three cultures—the culture of psychoanalysis, the culture of the modern NHS, and the culture of the Criminal Justice System. Each culture emphasizes different priorities and methods of evaluation: psychoanalysis focuses on unconscious processes and intrapsychic change, the NHS emphasizes accountability, monitoring and evaluation of interventions, and the need for meaningful and valid outcome research, whereas the Criminal Justice System highlights punishment, deterrence, and the reduction of recidivism. The Portman occupies an ambiguous position that attempts to bridge these different cultures and must allow for individuals within the clinic to locate themselves at different points within this matrix.

At the time of writing, the project is still in its infancy, and the group is as yet not running at full capacity. However, patients previously thought to be unreachable are attending, participating in treatment, and learning to tolerate and respect different points of view.

References

APA (1994). *Diagnostic and Statistical Manual of Mental Disorders* (4th edition, text revision). Washington, DC: American Psychiatric Association, 2000.

Baron-Cohen, S. (2005). The empathizing system: A revision of the 1994 model of the mind reading system. In: B. J. Ellis & D. F. Bjorklund (Eds.), *Origins of the Social Mind: Evolutionary Psychology and Child Development* (pp. 468–492). New York: Guilford Press.

Barry, C. T., Frick, P. J., DeShazo, T. M., McCoy, M. G., Ellis, M., & Loney, B. R. (2000). The importance of callous-unemotional traits for expanding the concept of psychopathy to children. *Journal of Abnormal Psychology, 109:* 335–340.

Bateman, A., & Fonagy, P. (2004). *Psychotherapy for Borderline Personality Disorder: Mentalization-Based Treatment.* Oxford: Oxford University Press.

Bateman, A., & Fonagy, P. (2006). *Mentalization-Based Treatment for Borderline Personality Disorder: A Practical Guide.* Oxford: Oxford University Press.

Bateman, A., & Fonagy, P. (2008). Co-morbid antisocial and borderline personality disorders: Mentalization-based treatment. *Journal of Clinical Psychology, 64* (2): 181–194.

Bateman, A., & Fonagy, P. (2011). Antisocial personality disorder. In: A. Bateman & P. Fonagy (Eds.), *Mentalizing in Mental Health Practice* (pp. 357–378). Washington, DC: American Psychiatric Publishing.

Bion, W. R. (1959). Attacks on linking. *International Journal of Psychoanalysis, 40:* 308–315. Also in: *Second Thoughts.* London: Karnac, 1984.

Bion, W. R. (1961). *Experiences in Groups.* London: Tavistock.

Bion, W. R. (1962). *Learning from Experience.* London: Karnac, 1984.

Britton, R. (1989). The missing link: Parental sexuality in the Oedipus complex. In: J. Steiner (Ed.), *The Oedipus Complex Today: Clinical Implications* (pp. 83–101). London: Karnac.

Cleckley, H. (1941). *The Mask of Sanity.* St Louis, MI: Mosby.

Coid, J., Yang, M., Tyrer, P., Roberts, A., & Ullrich, S. (2006). Prevalence and correlates of personality disorder in Great Britain. *British Journal of Psychiatry, 188:* 423–431.

DoH (1999). *Managing Dangerous People with Severe Personality Disorder: Proposals for Policy Development.* Joint Home Office/DoH Report. London: Home Office and Department of Health.

DoH (2003). *Personality Disorder: No Longer a Diagnosis of Exclusion.* London: Department of Health.

DoH (2009). *The Bradley Report: Lord Bradley's Review of People with Mental Health Problems or Learning Disabilities in the Criminal Justice System.* London: Department of Health. Available at: www.dh.gov.uk/en/Publicationsandstatistics/Publications/PublicationsPolicyAndGuidance/DH_098694

Dolan, B., & Coid, J. (1993). Summary of findings and recommendations for future research. In: B. Dolan & J. Coid (Eds.), *Psychopathic and Antisocial Personality Disorders*. London: Gaskell.

D'Silva, K., Duggan, C., & McCarthy, J. (2004). Does treatment really make psychopaths worse? A review of the evidence. *Journal of Personality Disorders, 18:* 163–177.

Duggan, C., Adams, A., McCarthy, L., Fenton, M., Lee, T., Binks, C., et al. (2006). *Systemic Review of the Effectiveness of the Pharmacological and Psychological Treatments of Those with Personality Disorder*. Commissioned by NHS National Programme on Forensic Mental Health Research and Development. Available at: www.liv.ac.uk/fmhweb/ MRD%2012%2033%20Final%20Report.pdf

Fonagy, P., & Bateman, A. (2010). A brief history of mentalization-based treatment and its roots in psychoanalytic theory and practice. In: M. B. Heller & S. Pollett (Eds.), *The Work of Psychoanalysts in the Public Health Sector* (pp. 156–176). London: Routledge.

Fonagy, P., Moran, G., & Target, M. (1993). Aggression and the psychological self. *International Journal of Psychoanalysis, 74:* 471–486.

Fonagy, P., Steele, M., Steele, H., Moran, G. S., & Higgitt, A. C. (1991). The capacity for understanding mental states: The reflective self in parent and child and its significance for security of attachment. *Infant Mental Health Journal, 12:* 201–218.

Fonagy, P., & Target, M. (1995). Understanding the violent patient: The use of the body and the role of the father. *International Journal of Psychoanalysis, 76:* 487–501.

Fonagy, P., & Target, M. (1996). Playing with reality: I. Theory of mind and the normal development of psychic reality. *International Journal of Psychoanalysis, 77:* 217–233.

Fonagy, P., & Target, M. (2000). Playing with reality: III. The persistence of dual psychic reality in borderline patients. *International Journal of Psychoanalysis, 81* (5): 853–874.

Fonagy, P., & Target, M. (2007). Playing with reality: IV. A theory of external reality rooted in intersubjectivity. *International Journal of Psychoanalysis, 88* (4): 917–937.

Foulkes, S. (1948). *Introduction to Group Analytic Psychotherapy*. London: Karnac, 1983.

Freud, S. (1916d). Some character types met with in psychoanalysis. *Standard Edition, 14*.

Frodi, A., Dernevik, M., Sepa, A., Philipson, J., & Bragesio, M. (2001). Current attachment representations of incarcerated offenders varying in degree of psychopathy. *Attachment and Human Development, 3:* 269–283.

Gabbard, G. (2005). *Psychodynamic Psychiatry in Clinical Practice* (4th edition). Washington, DC: American Psychiatric Press.

Gabbard, G., & Coyne, L. (1987). Predictors of response of antisocial patients to hospital treatment. *Hospital and Community Psychiatry, 38:* 1181–1185.

Gilligan, J. (1996). *Violence: Our Deadliest Epidemic and Its Causes.* New York: Grosset/Putnam.

Glasser, M. (1998). On violence: A preliminary communication. *International Journal of Psychoanalysis, 79:* 887–902.

Hare, R. D. (1991). *Manual for the Psychopathy Checklist.* Toronto: Multihealth Systems.

Hare, R. D. (2003). *Manual for the Psychopathy Checklist–Revised* (2nd edition). Toronto: Multihealth Systems.

Harris, G. T., Rice, M. E., & Cormier, C. A. (1991). Psychopathy and violent recidivism. *Law and Human Behaviour, 15:* 625–637.

Harris, G. T., Rice, M. E., & Cormier, C. A. (1994). Psychopaths: Is a therapeutic community therapeutic? *Therapeutic Communities, 15:* 283–299.

Home Office (2006). *Violent Crime Overview, Homicide and Gun Crime 2004/2005.* London: Home Office Research, Development and Statistics Directorate.

Jones, M. (1952). *A Study of Therapeutic Communities.* London: Tavistock.

Levinson, A., & Fonagy, P. (2004). Offending and attachment: The relationship between interpersonal awareness and offending in a prison population with psychiatric disorder. *Canadian Journal of Psychoanalysis, 12:* 225–251.

Livesley, W. J. (2004). Introduction to the special feature on recent progress in the treatment of personality disorder. *Journal of Personality Disorder, 18:* 1–2.

Lynam, D. R., & Gudonis, L. (2005). The development of psychopathy. *Annual Review of Clinical Psychopathy, 1:* 381–407.

McGauley, G., Adshead, G., & Sarkar, S. (2007). Psychotherapy of psychopathic disorders. In: A. Felthouse & H. Sass (Eds.), *The International Handbook of Psychopathic Disorders and the Law: Diagnosis and Treatment, Vol. 1.* (pp. 449–466). Chichester: John Wiley.

Meloy, J. R. (1992). *Violent Attachments.* Northvale, NJ: Jason Aronson.

Meloy, J. R. (1995). Antisocial personality disorder. In: G. O. Gabbard (Ed.), *Treatments of Psychiatric Disorders, Vol. 2* (2nd edition, pp. 2273–2290). Washington, DC: American Psychiatric Press.

Ministry of Justice (2008). *Arrests for Recorded Crime (Notifiable Offences) and the Operation of Certain Police Powers under PACE England and Wales 2006/07*. Available at: www.justice.gov.uk/docs/arrests-recorded-crime-engl-wales-2006–07.pdf

NICE (2009). *Antisocial Personality Disorder: Treatment, Management and Prevention*. NICE Clinical Guideline 77. London: National Institute for Health and Clinical Excellence. Available at: http://guidance.nice.org.uk/CG77

Ogloff, J. R. P., Wong, S., & Greenwood, A. (1990). Treating criminal psychopaths in a therapeutic community program. *Behavioural Sciences and the Law, 8:* 181–190.

Patrick, C. (Ed.) (2006). *Handbook of Psychopathy*. New York: Guilford Press.

Salekin, R. (2002). Psychopathy and therapeutic pessimism: Clinical lore or clinical reality. *Clinical Psychology Review, 22:* 79–112.

Saville, E., & Rumney, D. (1992). *"Let Justice Be Done!": A History of the ISTD*. London: Institute for the Study and Treatment of Delinquency.

Tardiff, K. (2003). Violence: Causes and non-psychopharmacological treatment. In: R. Rosner (Ed.), *Principles and Practice of Forensic Psychiatry* (2nd edition). London: Arnold.

Target, M., & Fonagy, P. (1996). Playing with reality II: The development of psychic reality from a developmental perspective. *International Journal of Psychoanalysis, 77:* 459–479.

Torgensen, S., Kringlen, E., & Cramer, V. (2001). The prevalence of personality disorders in a community sample. *Archives of General Psychiatry, 58:* 590–596.

van IJzendoorn, M. H., Feldbrugge, J. T. T. M., Derks, F. C. H., de Ruiter, C., Verhagen, M. F. M., Philipse, M. W. G., et al. (1997). Attachment representations of personality-disordered criminal offenders. *American Journal of Orthopsychiatry, 67:* 449–459.

Viding, E., Larsson, H., & Jones, A. P. (2008). Review: Quantitative genetic studies of antisocial behaviour. *Philosophical Transactions of the Royal Society of London B: Biological Sciences, 363:* 2519–2527.

Webster, C. D., Douglas, K. S., Eaves, D., & Hart, S. T. (1997). *HCR-20: Assessing Risk for Violence, Version 2*. Vancouver: Mental Health, Law and Policy Institute, Simon Fraser University.

WHO (1992). *International Statistical Classification of Diseases and Related Health Problems* (10th revision, ICD-10). Geneva: World Health Organization.

Winnicott, D. W. (1954). Metapsychological and clinical aspects of regression within the psychoanalytic set-up. In: *Through Paediatrics to Psychoanalysis*. London: Hogarth Press, 1975. Reprinted London: Karnac, 1992.

Winnicott, D. W. (1956). The anti-social tendency. In: D. W. Winnicott (Ed.), *Through Paediatrics to Psychoanalysis* (pp. 306–315). London: Hogarth Press, 1975. Reprinted London: Karnac, 1992.

CHAPTER NINE

Where Internet was, there ego shall be: community and well-being in the digital world

Richard Graham

Over the past 20 years rapid developments in technology have radically changed the ways individuals communicate or form groups and communities: they can now spend almost half of their waking time online, communicating with each other. There is now an unprecedented capacity for any individual with access to the Internet to be in contact with a multitude of others and communicate ideas and beliefs to an entire world. However, while this creates a powerful opportunity to promote change, without a stable capacity for judgement there is a risk of causing harm as well as improving a sense of well-being. This chapter aims to explore the opportunities afforded by the digital revolution in promoting contact between individuals and establishing communities that can have a therapeutic effect. The emphasis is thus both on mental well-being and mental distress and how these may be attended to in online communities.

This chapter describes how psychoanalysis afforded a deeper understanding of mankind's group behaviour, which led to an appreciation of how communities can function. The work and ideas of Wilfred Bion are explored, particularly those that emerged when he worked as an Army psychiatrist during the Second World War and observed how a community can be mobilized to find solutions to its own problems and consequently improve its sense of well-being. The latter part of the chapter describes how the Tavistock and Portman NHS Foundation Trust, recognizing the opportunities of the digital world, has established a partnership with an online well-being service, Big White Wall, to promote the well-being of its members, through the facilitation of its community activities and positive relationships.

The power of community

At the close of the nineteenth century, the emergence of psychoanalysis in Europe could be thought of as a continuation of responses to both the Industrial Revolution and the greater shift of the global population to urban living. Freud's interest in individual psychology was accompanied by considerations of group psychology and the processes of civilization. His thinking was often tinged with an acute awareness of how urban life created significant difficulties for anyone living within it. It is perhaps not just coincidence that one of the first major works on group psychology, by Gustav Le Bon—*La psychologie des Foules*—was published in 1895, the same year as Freud's "Project for a Scientific Psychology" (1950 [1895]). The influence of urban life on post-industrialized man was salient to the ideas both men were developing. Freud's own work on the subject, *Group Psychology and the Analysis of the Ego* (Freud, 1921c), draws more on the later phenomena of the First World War and informed works on life within groups, notably *Civilization and its Discontents* (Freud, 1930a), which highlighted the problems not so much of civilized man as of urban man. Inevitably, the impact of the First World War and the dramatic rise in urban living lent these theories a negative quality that excluded the positives that may also result from group living in urban environments.

In England, in 1920, the establishment of the Tavistock Clinic by Hugh Crichton-Miller was intended to be a response to the ills of society and an attempt to assist with them. In Henry Dicks' 1970 volume celebrating the 50th anniversary of the Tavistock, he suggests that while the early work was informed by individual psychology, the greater vision was to realize the importance of "What was going on in the social groups in which the individual lived as well as the factors that his own development had formed within himself" (Farrer, 1970, p. ix).

While it was an awareness of functional illness that led Crichton-Miller to abandon general practice and establish Bowden House in 1911, it was his experience of treating soldiers, first during the First World War and then in its aftermath, as they returned to civilian life, that led to foundation of the Tavistock Clinic. The devastation of the First World War had confirmed the importance of psychological stress upon the individual but also the crucial importance of group psychology.

Wilfred Bion, a psychiatrist with first-hand experience of the war, would later absorb much from the early work of the Clinic and take the problem of the "felt social need" as a considerable task to engage with.

Prior to the establishment of any therapeutic community, health experiments led by biologists and physiologists in Peckham had some surprising social outcomes, which would inform later social experiments:

> The "Peckham Experiment" described an unintentional therapeutic community that had grown up in Peckham, South London in the 1930s. It arose from an attempt . . . to monitor a number of health related factors over the long term. The subjects were local families prepared to . . . take part in a program of regular tests. Originally a swimming pool was the main draw—only family units could join. While fulfilling its part of the bargain in relation to the tests, over time the community developed a life of its own. [Bridger, 1990, p. 76]

By the 1940s, against the background of the Second World War, discussions between Wilfred Bion and his former analyst John Rickman led to a revolutionary suggestion as to how a mental health service might be organized, influenced no doubt by Bion's repeated experiences of the harm caused by authoritarian leadership. Taking its name from the hospital in Sheffield where Rickman was working, Bion wrote *The Wharnecliffe Memorandum* (of which no copy seems to exist), in which he suggested a very different model of treatment to the psychiatric care offered to inpatients at that time:

> One of the most important achievements of social psychiatry during World War II was the discovery of the therapeutic community. The idea of using all the relationships and activities of a residential psychiatric centre to aid the therapeutic task was first put forward by Wilfred Bion in 1940. . . . It entailed a radical change in staff/

> patient relations which produced a figure/ground reversal in the
> traditional authoritarian hospital. In order to achieve active patient
> participation in treatment, power was to be distributed away from
> its monopolization by the doctor and shared by other staff and
> patients in appropriate ways. [Bridger, 1990, p. 68]

Unfortunately there was too great a resistance to this transformation
of the power relationships within the Wharnecliffe Hospital for any
change to occur, but the Memorandum did inform further wartime
developments. First, Bion, along with other pre-war Tavistock psychiatrists, developed a process to assist the recruitment of officers
within the army, using a model of leaderless groups. These groups,
along with psychological tests, proved very successful in identifying
those who had the knowledge, skills, and leadership capacities to take
on the role of officer during the war. The method became established
in the War Office Selection Boards, which then successfully spread to
other services.

But the demands of the Second World War created a further problem in relation to servicemen suffering combat stress and the needs
for the nation to continue fighting a war. The need on this occasion
was to reduce the "neurotic behaviour" of the soldiers at the Northfield Military Hospital in Birmingham, so that they were then able to
function at a more effective level, either in civilian life or through a
return to army activities. As at Wharnecliffe, Bion had been concerned
about the way in which the hospital was structured, in terms of its
resources and of where power was located. His challenge to the model
of medical authority so dominant at the time is striking:

> Time and again treatment appears to be, in the broadest sense,
> sedative; sedative for doctors and patients alike. Occupational
> therapy meant helping keep the patients occupied—usually on
> a kindergarten level. Some patients had individual interviews;
> a few, usually the more spectacular, were dosed with hypnotics.
> Sometimes a critic might be forgiven for wondering whether these
> were intended to enable the doctor to go to sleep.
>
>   It thus seemed necessary to bring the atmosphere of the psy-
> chiatric hospital into closer relationship with the functions it ought
> to fulfil. [Bion, quoted in Bridger, 1990, p. 70]

Bion, working with Rickman, established a model of treatment with
apparently very few demands. First, the group of soldiers were asked
to attend a daily parade and exercise; apart from that, they could
organize themselves into groups to undertake activities of whatever

nature they chose. These included handicrafts, swimming, cinema, dancing, and football, and all of these interests could be pursued without question or criticism. The soldiers subsequently raised a number of problems with Bion, notably concerning the "80%" of soldiers who were described as being "work-shy". Bion refused to take responsibility for this problem and, instead, gave it back to the community as one that was common to many societies and unlikely to be resolved by the simple use of punishment. The soldiers were asked to explore and consider this problem further. Bion's refusal to take on the role of psychiatrist in the manner that the soldiers expected of him had a very powerful effect. The project only lasted six weeks, but by then there had been such an improvement in the majority of soldiers that they felt able to re-engage with the military role. However, the fear and chaos created in this process was so intolerable to the wider hospital staff, who still clung to the traditional medical model, that Bion and Rickman were dismissed.

Harold Bridger, who developed this model further in the Second Northfield Experiment, believed that the extent of success Bion achieved in the six weeks demonstrated the validity of his hypothesis and of the power of community. However, the destabilization of the wider system indicated that the introduction of change processes necessitated a search for a common purpose and methods, plus a forum in which a collegiate climate could grow.

The Northfield Experiments led to a significant change in thinking and, later, to important developments in the civil resettlement units, which were set up for repatriated prisoners of war. Two years after Northfield, Bion was posted to a War Office Selection Board in Surrey. By this time, near the end of the war, the redeployment of officers had become necessary. Officers were referred from both the United Kingdom and abroad and attended voluntarily to

> Sort out their problems and redefine their roles and careers as temporary or regular soldiers. There was a lot of depression about becoming surplus, reduced in rank, having become a misfit; confusion and anxiety about the future; ignorance of opportunities and loss of confidence in abilities. [Trist, 1985, p. 20]

Bion understood this in the context of *transition points*, which created tensions and stresses that could be used to enhance personal growth and learning. Led by regimental rather than medical control, the Board functioned such that

There was no division of intake into patients and non-patients. No one had to be labelled as neurotic or normal, or think of himself as suffering from a "disease".

He next instituted two simple but fundamental principles. There was no fixed length of stay; anyone could come back on request. The role of the unit was to be a "depot ship". He wanted it perceived as a persisting, reliable, and accessible "good project". The degree to which one made use of its resources was determined by oneself. [Trist, 1985, p. 20]

In addition to empowering the officers, it will be very apparent that Bion's empathy and sensitivity to the anxieties of the returning officers established a setting as free of stigma as it may have been possible to achieve at the time. The Board in Surrey, in addition to the Northfield Experiments, set in motion a process that for a while was able to challenge the conventional delivery of services, so that they could both involve users and be made more accessible through this involvement of service users.

It is somewhat disappointing to note, almost 70 years later, that many of the developments made during the Second World War were only partially sustained, though some processes, such as increasing user involvement, are now finding their place again in modern healthcare services. There are perhaps two consequences to the return to a medical model service. First, repeated studies show that many suffering from mental health difficulties either find it difficult to access services or choose not to. In the Adult Psychiatric Morbidity Survey of 2007 (NHS IC, 2007), only a quarter of the 15% of the population suffering from anxiety and depression were receiving any treatment, and if they were, it was usually in the form of medication. Over a third of those who reported having attempted suicide did not seek help. Only a fifth of the 9% of women suffering from an eating disorder were receiving treatment. Other studies highlight that those from minority groups are reluctant to engage in treatment and do not find it sensitive to their needs. It is with some discomfort that the "felt social need" of the early years of the twentieth century is still very much with us. The dominance of a medical model remains in most settings; despite various policy initiatives, it is difficult—as Bion found—to involve everyone in the process, when concerns over risk and governance reinforce a need for an authoritarian medical leadership. However, the "lessons learnt" by Bion have left an important mark on the work of the Tavistock Clinic, especially the ongoing belief in the power of the group, which can be discerned in recent developments in online therapeutic interventions, as I now describe.

Health and happiness in the modern world

One area where there has been a rather different, "non-medical" approach is in the field of mental well-being. It has perhaps become a more urgent problem to understand what promotes health and happiness in the modern world. The understanding of positive mental health has become an important and influential approach both to promoting mental well-being and to reducing mental disorder; the two are independent in that it is possible to have a high level of mental well-being despite having a severe or enduring mental disorder. While therapeutic work may reduce distress or promote development, the current research on mental well-being does suggest that there are activities or aspects to our lives that promote well-being independently—much as a good level of physical health can be achieved through diet, exercise, and avoiding high levels of noxious substances.

Keyes (2007) categorized the 13 elements of flourishing or positive mental well-being into three groups: (1) *emotional well-being* includes a positive affect and satisfaction with the quality of life; (2) *psychological well-being* includes self-acceptance, personal growth, having a purpose in life, and having a sense of autonomy, mastery of the environment, and positive relations to others; (3) *social well-being* includes those aspects of social experience such as social acceptance, social contribution, and social integration. Of the 13 elements, a significant number will relate to the community in which the individual lives and will therefore require a different approach from one focused upon the individual.

In 1986, the World Health Organization described how individual orientated interventions may reduce the health hazards of the individual, but the very significant environmental hazards, such as a lack of good nutrition, housing, employment, or education, require a community-orientated intervention. Given that some of these factors require human resources as much as material ones, the manner in which a community is able to organize itself will play a profound role here. Indeed, the Scottish Mental Health and Well-being Adult

Indicators emphasize that a great many factors that promote well-being are dependent upon inclusion and participation in a safe, supportive community, in which discrimination and violence are minimal and the opportunities for learning and employment significant.

The New Economics Foundation was commissioned by the government's Foresight Mental Capital and Wellbeing Project (GO-Science, 2008) in order to recommend the five activities for achieving well-being—the equivalent of the five portions of fruit and vegetables that were to be consumed each day to maintain good physical health. They are:

⊳ Connect: connect with those around you, including family and friends.

⊳ Be active: go for a regular walk or run.

⊳ Take notice: be mindful of what is going on around you and savour each moment.

⊳ Keep learning: challenge yourself to try something new.

⊳ Give: this can be as simple as smiling, saying thank you, or volunteering.

These five activities may seem simplistic, even patronizing. Yet they are based on research into people who are flourishing and offer an evidence-based contribution to how we can improve our state of mind and well-being.

It would be unfair to those trying to improve the well-being of the population to assume that the five ways are in any way a substitute for health interventions that reduce mental distress. Indeed, a cornerstone of the well-being programme has been to increase access to psychological therapies, such that they can be accessed at an earlier level of distress or disorder, and suffering can consequently be reduced.

The issues of poverty and poor housing, as a product of urban living, continue to echo the questions that preoccupied Freud and many others in the last century: living in close proximity to others does not in any way predict a positive quality to community life, which, as indicated by the "Peckham Experiment" in the 1930s, has to be worked for. It could indeed be argued that psychoanalysis and subsequent psychological therapies have arisen to attend to the individual health hazards of post-industrial life. However, there are inevitable limitations if the focus of interventions is only on the individual, when what happens within the community is a powerful agent of change. Awareness of individual and community processes is both necessary and requires "binocular vision" at strategic and policy levels. Furthermore, it has been recognized that current services only reach a fraction of those in need of intervention, and for many there remains considerable stigma attached to seeking help. At this point access to psychological therapy, whatever its type and limitations, is a problem not just of availability, but of it being accessed in a way that helps the individual feel relatively comfortable. The quest is therefore to find a method in which users can access a service in a manner that is entirely under their control.

The digital revolution: engaging with the new world

The dissemination of the research findings regarding well-being, and what promotes it, has become increasingly important in current society. The new world of digital technologies facilitates wider access to such knowledge but offers little direction in supporting its use, without either personal recommendation or community support for it. In recognition of this, and in following its earliest goals, the Tavistock and Portman NHS Foundation Trust sought to increase access to its own knowledge of well-being and development and embraced the possibilities of the digital world in a creative partnership with an online mental well-being service, Big White Wall. This online community allows previously unimaginable opportunities for imparting knowledge that could influence the well-being of any individual member. The resources within any community are such that if they can be mobilized, through a redistribution of power, in the form of information, from current structures, they can have enormous potential. This potential requires, however, that the ensuing chaos from this redistribution can be contained.

Developments in information technology, and more recently in social media, are not simply naturalistic evolutions of technology but necessary developments to combat the deficits inherent in urban living today. It is beyond the scope of this chapter to outline in detail the evolution of the Internet, which has its roots in military and technological research into computer networks of the late 1950s. It is worth noting however, that the current form—the World Wide

Web—was invented just over 20 years ago by Tim Berners-Lee. The last decade has offered much greater access through the establishing of broadband services, which can now facilitate a much greater contact between those using the Internet.

If it is extraordinary to consider that it is only just over 20 years since the World Wide Web was invented, it is perhaps even more extraordinary that the more recent developments in social media have come about within the past 5–6 years. Social media are media used for social interaction, using highly accessible and scalable publishing techniques. World Wide Web–based technologies turn communication into interactive dialogues. Andreas Kaplan and Michael Haenlein (2010) also define social media as "a group of Internet-based applications that build on the ideological and technological foundations of Web 2.0, which allows the creation and exchange of user-generated content". This rather dry definition gives little indication of the pulsating enthusiasm with which the opportunities of social networking have been embraced so rapidly by the global population. Indeed, at this point it is anticipated that there will be an even more dramatic use of social media in countries that are developing rapidly, such as China, Brazil, and India, with little suggestion of any slowdown in take-up.

The most frequently used platforms at this time are Facebook, Twitter, and MySpace, with specific platforms such as YouTube and Flickr being used for the sharing of video and photographic material, respectively. The rise in the use of Facebook has been so extraordinarily rapid and extensive—far eclipsing the take-up of earlier technologies such as radio and television—that some have questioned whether it should be considered a utility and subject to regulation. Twitter, a platform for communicating brief messages of no more than 140 characters, has seen as fast a rise in utilization: despite being only four years old, it currently (at the time of writing) has 175 million users globally, though this is dwarfed by Facebook's current 800 million users worldwide.

A significant part of the social media revolution is the manner in which even relatively recent modes of communication, such as email, are now in decline, as the opportunities for instant messaging and its creation of a sense of near-continuous contact with an individual, group, or community have grown. The power of a community to mobilize its resources—such as skills, knowledge—can now occur at a global level, and previous considerations as to the size of a large group or even crowd, inevitably limited by corporeal realities and physical space, are no longer an obstacle. These are some of the aspects to this new world that need further consideration.

In addition to one's physical reality, rooted in bodily experience and the psychic reality of the mind, there is now a third, digital reality in which we also exist as substantially as in the other worlds. The digital world has been compared to a city that you may not know well, and in which you may have little sense of what is safe and what is risky. It is unfortunately—putting aside those risks related to others exploiting personal information—a world in which actions can be achieved very quickly, at the push of a button, whether we are in states of intoxication or sober, excited, enraged, or calm. It is unfortunate that the resulting consequences can be devastating—such as the rise of online gambling and illegal pornography. The speed of communications and actions is such that Freud's (1911b) formulation of thought as "trial action", located between impulse and action, barely occurs as impulses find their satisfactions, in particular and largely visual ways, immediately. Given the possibilities of making public on the Internet any area of interest, no matter how positive or perverse, it is possible to find material relating to almost any conscious and unconscious fantasy or undertake actions that can barely be dreamed of. The possibilities of intrusion, impersonation, and secret activity create considerable risks.

Recent research (Moreno et al., 2009) relating to the social media site MySpace revealed a striking overrepresentation on the individual profiles of young people of material relating to violence, substance misuse, and sexual activity. Primitive or gang-like behaviours took precedence over more thoughtful or sensitive contact, and the information itself was largely unregulated by any adults. The very scale of the World Wide Web makes it extremely difficult to regulate or moderate such processes—as if the digital world, in its current state, lacks the type of thoughtful, cooperative leadership and authority that was present in the Northfield Experiments, no matter how disruptive or chaotic they may have been.

Unfortunately, whatever the risks, the digital world in which many young people and adults are spending increasing amounts of their time in the pursuit of a feeling of inclusion or connectedness and community is creating difficulties in relation to the new world. Most obvious is the all too common phenomenon of cyberbullying, where savage attacks on another occur freely and repeatedly. More disturbing is the phenomenon of cyberstalking, where noxious messages are sent so frequently each day that the tumult of them violates the victim and renders him or her helpless. In addition, false information posted on various sites, or through impersonation and messaging, may have further catastrophic consequences. Current cases show that the perpetrators of such acts are not the technologically astute young people one might expect: in some cases they appear to be relatively ordinary individuals in later life enacting the most sadistic phantasies in the secret quietness of their homes.

These concerns should, however, not blunt our engagement with the possibilities of this new phenomenon, in which the sharing of information redistributes power to the occupants of this world in an unprecedented manner. Political processes and legal procedures aimed at the restriction of information can be bypassed in the pursuit of democracy, even if we are learning that the limitations of privacy in the digital world are not without their own risks. Users of services can share information; protest groups can form easily, grow rapidly using platforms such as Facebook, and subsequently challenge the establishment. While this undoubtedly can create an air of threat and chaos, there is considerable power to mobilize communities within this world—for good as much as ill.

Big White Wall:
where ego shall be

It does not seem fanciful, at this point in time, to consider the World Wide Web and its activities as having an uncanny similarity to the Unconscious as described by Freud. There are websites that are facsimiles of unconscious phantasies, including sexual and sadistic phantasies; impulse-, sensation-, or pleasure-driven activities are in ascendance. While considerable thought and research time is devoted to the development of technology, it is much more difficult to represent a credible thinking function online—that is, to maintain a capacity for discrimination and judgement, not in terms of content but in terms of processes or functionality. This may be partly due to the sheer novelty of the technology, which stirs both excitement and anxiety in those trying to understand it, but it undoubtedly also relates to commercial interests, as with the discovery of any new world. The response of authoritarian control and regulation is often a result, or an almost mindless acceptance, when either risks or opportunities are exaggerated to a near-extreme degree. It has been a struggle to promote balanced points of view online, where thought and consideration can be brought to bear on the very real opportunities of engaging with individuals and groups in our societies.

In 2008, the Tavistock and Portman NHS Trust, in partnership with Big White Wall, was able to offer an early intervention online for those experiencing psychological distress. It was apparent that at that time the site offered an unusually supportive environment in which the resources of the community could be drawn upon to support a range of therapeutic interventions, both safely and anonymously. The founder, Jenny Hyatt, had established a community in which the good will and support between its users could facilitate recovery or development using online arts materials, writing in groups (the theme of which is defined by the person starting it), and self-help material to promote all areas of well-being, including emotional health, physical well-being, relationships, and life skills.

According to Jenny Hyatt, a key aspect to having established this culture is the motive for going online: users of Big White Wall go online primarily with the intention of finding help and support, and to be supportive of others. In that sense, the community is less interested in the perverse distractions of violence or sexual content that are found on other sites, and there is a shared belief in a good object that can offer something. This is often represented by its founder, though at other times simply by the site itself, and the empty space of the Wall. At times this aspect of the community can be profoundly moving.

During the early discussions with Big White Wall, it became apparent that the opportunities of the site and peer-to-peer support were not entirely meeting the needs of those using the site. A survey of members of the site indicated that they felt they needed more than just support, and they made a request for more in-depth therapeutic interventions, and also that the facilitators of the site (Wall Guides) should have some therapeutic training. This feedback created the opportunity for a partnership, where the knowledge and skills of the Tavistock Clinic could be brought into this new world, though modified and made accessible to a much wider community than could reach the building. For those using the site, it was also hoped that they could access help earlier, no matter where they were living, and thus might be able to minimize the chances of long-term suffering.

At this point it might be helpful to describe what Big White Wall currently offers its members, and what actually happens when someone accesses the site. After a registration process, the new member is asked to complete a brief questionnaire that identifies severe or enduring mental health problems and alerts the Wall Guides to their level of vulnerability. The member then enters the full site and is shown a range possibilities. This experience itself can let us know something of the inner life of a member, through understanding what their individual experience has been, and also through considering this in the context of acknowledging how comfortable—or not—they feel in the online environment. Knowing about and thus navigating between the options available does take some time to learn, but once familiar, users are free to choose how much they engage with any activity or how much time they spend in different areas. This does not eliminate a feeling of exposure in the first moments, though familiarity with social media platforms and online forums might limit that. To begin with, a person may just observe what is going on and slowly decide how much he or she wishes to engage. Indeed, it is so completely under his or her control that one can see that the site has many parallels with the "depot ship" service for returning officers, developed by Bion at the close of the Second World War. Wall Guides will welcome any new member and offer to answer any questions. In the early days, someone may only engage with the Wall Guides, though the effectiveness of the site largely resides in community or group activities.

While there is written information on many areas of mental well-being on the site, identified as "Useful Stuff", other areas are more interactive. A range of standard mental health measures on all common mental disorders are available as members complete "Tests" and then reflect upon their results. The site will create a thoughtful and evidence-based response for any score and offer suggestions for next steps. Questionnaires can be completed whenever desired and even repeated over time, creating a personal thinking space in which to reflect upon an area that troubles the user. This could relate to trauma, or drug and alcohol use, or an eating disorder, and whatever the result of a test, there are only suggestions as to how to take the issue further, which may be that hour, that week, or in six months' time. A fundamental aspect of the site is that advice-giving or persuasion is neither acceptable nor tolerated from anyone, such that the site can be perceived as neither intrusive nor controlling, and members may find their own solutions. This fortuitously avoids the pitfalls of any treatment, which can so easily repeat traumatic experiences of helplessness and intrusion.

While the questionnaires add a degree of self-determined interactivity, by far the most lively and supportive aspect of the site is in its community, where users may create "Bricks", with images and text, or participate in "Talkabouts", which follow a theme defined by the person who established the Talkabout. Talkabout themes can be as broad as feeling "Trapped", or "Coping with aggressive people" to "My day in six words" or "Weather anxieties". Some discussions develop more life than others, depending upon who is accessing the site at the time, and the facilitation from the Wall Guides comes with a "light touch"—risk management of content is discreet. Indeed, the users are often vocal at any perceived attempts to be "nannied", though careful guidelines for safety are in place, such that the most vulnerable can feel that they are supported.

A brief illustration of the kind of exchanges that take place on the site may be helpful at this point.

Community Talkabout

A new member of the site created a Talkabout the content of which suggested he had worked within the police force. The member felt angry and distressed by the sheer impact upon him of some traumatic experiences, but also that he felt betrayed by the senior managers, who, he felt, had lost their way. The member was very anxious that his state of mind could become worse and that he would not be able to return to work. This itself created a huge dilemma as to whether or not to disclose what was so troubling to him; the anonymity of the site offered some cover. Nightmares interrupted sleep, and now even small incidents reported on the television caused distress. What was more difficult was that, unlike some colleagues, he had never suffered any physical injury in the course of duty and "posted" that he felt bad about "moaning". The last words were: "No one to turn to."

The Guides, alerted to this new member's distress, thought that it was important to offer support, but their dilemma was how long the community should be allowed to respond to its own members before a Guide intervened. During this deliberation, another member posted a response:

"Turning somewhere. Not easy.... I drink to fall over to stop falling. You?"

The empathy, even understanding, afforded at this moment reduced the new member's feeling of isolation and created the hope that further communication might help him.

Another member of the community, with all of its different personalities and experiences, could find the words to help the new member feel included, with a poetry that a clinician might struggle to achieve. A small dialogue was established, perhaps of just the right size, but one that could progress to communication about nightmares, and the experiences before them.

The subtlety of interaction and sensitivity demonstrated towards other members is sometimes replaced by irritation, even confrontation, but, most of the time, the community can be mobilized sensitively by its members. One interesting dimension to the community is our growing understanding of how the online environment can be structured and shaped to offer differing levels of containment or security and therein have different levels of therapeutic possibility. The "street-level" quality of the Community Talkabouts allows for some discussion of difficulties, but closer contact between members is less common, as the interactions are so public. The anonymity of presenting oneself under the pseudonym of a username only helps so much, though it has been very successful in helping those who otherwise struggle to access services, including men and those from minority groups. The pseudonym—a self-created "username"—itself can say a great deal to the whole community, but it is in Group Talkabouts and Personal Talkabouts that members are able to establish a space that is more personal and private. Some preliminary experience of establishing therapeutic groups in a more private and boundaried space are very promising. This highlights how the Internet can be perceived as wild and open—again like the unconscious—if not structured in relation to privacy.

Moderator activity of the Wall Guides necessarily allows them some knowledge of the content of these personal and group spaces, to reduce the risk of members influencing each other adversely in unseen places. However, when a group has been established by a therapist, the associated reduced moderation by a Guide in relation to that group also lends it a more potent therapeutic capacity. It is this process of understanding how to establish a therapeutic setting in an online environment that is proving to be one of the most fascinating and exciting areas of current work. It seems entirely possible that when our understanding of the factors that create a therapeutic setting are advanced, the possibilities for therapeutic change could be considerable. It is certainly the case that the impact of online material can be very substantial, and at times traumatic, for all of us, which does indicate its considerable power to influence our psychology. Further questions regarding the process of material entering the mind through the eyes are also subject to investigation.

Another area for consideration and understanding relates to the creative activities, using visual arts, that are possible on the site. "Bricks", like Talkabouts, can be created completely by one member. The process of creation itself appears to have considerable potential to facilitate change, not just in terms of content, but as a mental process of creating a symbolic representation of a state of mind that one wishes to communicate. It is possible that so much online activity is largely a passive feeding of the mind—the illusion of being fed by a present object. As Melanie Klein noted in her work on the creative processes, "Infantile Anxiety Situations Reflected in a Work of Art and in the Creative Impulse" (1929), in addition to any self-expression, reparative trends in the self seek to restore or create through art that which is feared lost. Through the creative process, it becomes possible to restore an absent object in the inner world and feel more hopeful. The thinking and wish to communicate that may lie behind the creation of the Brick requires a higher level of mental activity and relatedness (even if the aim is to leave the viewer with unwanted feelings and thought) that itself is part of a journey to greater well-being; the mind is engaged at a deeper level. Uploaded onto the Wall, the Bricks can have a very powerful impact but also take their place in the community, where all members have the option of creating a Brick and sharing the Wall space. Personal development can also be charted through the Bricks created over time, creating a sense of time passing. Comments may be added, giving the background to a Brick which others can respond to. One member writes of this process:

"I was incredibly sceptical about this site, and also anxious, as I find it difficult to talk about my difficulties and did not want to appear to be an attention seeker. I was wrong to think in that way. Thank you for providing this safe space for me to jot down thoughts, feelings etc. as they come rather than having to wait to see a therapist. It is good to be able to share with the community, and know there are others out there with or who had similar problems and learn about how they have dealt with them; I feel much less isolated :-)"

This post identifies the start of a journey, which may lead to engagement in therapeutic work, perhaps face-to-face, when thinking and waiting are more manageable. The member may engage more actively in the community, discussing feelings at a deeper level, or may in one of the Group or Personal Spaces feel able to discuss more openly what troubles him or her. The current use, almost as a diary, to acknowledge to oneself what is on one's mind, has its value.

Concluding thoughts

It is moving to witness what can be achieved through the community, and how those in the most troubled states, on the verge of suicide, find help that supports them through a crisis. There is work to be done in terms of improving aspects of the site, including online therapeutic work, which is now under way. It may well be that the community has much greater power to effect change and improve well-being than through any individual encounter. It is a privilege for the Trust at this point to be guided through the digital era, in the hope of establishing a credible and effective presence that can be accessed by many hundreds of people, safely and even economically.

References

Bridger, H. (1990). The discovery of the therapeutic community: The Northfield experiments. In: E. Trist & H. Murray (Eds.), *The Social Engagement of Social Science, Vol. I: The Socio-Psychological Perspective*. London: Free Association Books.

Dicks, H. V. (1970). *Fifty Years of the Tavistock Clinic*. London: Routledge & Kegan Paul.

Farrer, L. (1970). Foreword. In: H. V. Dicks, *Fifty Years of the Tavistock Clinic*. London: Routledge & Kegan Paul.

Freud, S. (1911b). Formulations on the two principles of mental functioning. *Standard Edition, 12*.

Freud, S. (1921c). *Group Psychology and the Analysis of the Ego. Standard Edition, 18*: 69.

Freud, S. (1930a). *Civilization and Its Discontents. Standard Edition, 21*.

Freud, S. (1950 [1895]). Project for a scientific psychology. *Standard Edition, 1*.

GO-Science (2008). *Foresight Mental Capital and Wellbeing Project: Final Project Report*. London: The Government Office for Science.

Kaplan, A. M., & Haenlein, M. (2010). Users of the world, unite! The challenges and opportunities of Social Media. *Business Horizons, 53* (1): 59–68.

Keyes, C. (2007). Promoting and protecting mental health as flourishing: A complementary strategy for improving national mental health. *American Psychologist, 62*: 95–108.

Klein, M. (1929). Infantile anxiety situations reflected in a work of art and in the creative impulse. In: *Love, Guilt and Reparation and Other Works 1921–1945* (pp. 210–218). London: Hogarth Press, 1985.

Moreno, M. A., Parks, M. R., Zimmerman, F. J., Brito, T. E., & Christakis, D. A. (2009). Display of health risk behaviors on MySpace by adolescents: Prevalence and associations. *Archives of Pediatrics & Adolescent Medicine, 163* (1): 27–34.

NHS IC (2007). *Adult Psychiatric Morbidity in England 2007*. Leeds: NHS Information Centre for Health and Social Care. Available at: www.ic.nhs.uk/pubs

Trist, E. (1985). Working with Bion in the 1940s: The group decade. In: M. Pines (Ed.), *Bion and Group Psychotherapy*. London: Routledge & Kegan Paul.

CHAPTER TEN

Dynamic interpersonal therapy (DIT): developing a new intervention for depression

Alessandra Lemma, Mary Target, & Peter Fonagy

"Depression", a patient said, ". . . feels like wearing a beautifully embroidered black veil. I know I can't see things clearly through it, but I don't know that I could reveal myself to the world without it." This comment captures vividly the complexity of depression: it is a disabling condition, and yet the relationship an individual may have with it—that is, its function in the patient's psychic economy—may make the patient fearful of change and hence resistant to being helped.

Depression is a common and often complex condition that typically manifests early in life: 40% of depressed people experience a first episode by age 20 (Eaton et al., 2008). It interferes with social and occupational functioning, is associated with considerable morbidity, and carries a significant risk of mortality through suicide (Ustun, Ayuso-Mateos, Chatterji, Mathers, & Murray, 2004). Incomplete recovery and relapse are all too common. Following the first episode of major depression, people will go on to have at least one more episode (Kupfer, 1991), and the risk of further relapse rises sharply, to 70% and 90%, after the second and third episodes, respectively (Kupfer, 1991).

Its aetiology is not fully understood, but it is likely to be overdetermined by psychological, social, and biological processes (Fonagy, 2010; Goldberg, 2009; Malhi et al., 2009; Taylor, 2009). It is also common for depressed people to have a co-morbid psychiatric diagnosis, such as anxiety and various personality disorders (Kessler et al., 2003; Moffitt et al., 2007). Patients meeting criteria for a major depressive disorder are nine times more likely than chance to meet criteria for other conditions (Angst & Dobler-Mikola, 1985). Some 50–90% of patients with Axis I conditions also meet criteria for other Axis I or Axis II conditions (Westen, Novotny, & Thompson-Brenner, 2004).

Alongside the evident complexity of depression, an apparently simplistic approach has prevailed at the level of service provision within the public health sector, where the current emphasis on evidence-based practice has privileged cognitive behavioural therapy as the treatment of choice for depression. This "one-size-fits-all" approach to treatment has strongly marginalized psychoanalytic interventions. The superiority of CBT in this respect has been rightly questioned, not because it is not helpful to many depressed patients—it evidently is—but because it is not helpful to *all* depressed patients. Randomized controlled trials (RCTs) show that, as with all available treatments, a substantial minority of patients do not benefit sufficiently—around 50% responding adequately across treatments, with half of those losing gains over the following year (e.g. Roth & Fonagy, 2005). No single treatment has the answer for everyone, and a variety of approaches with some evidence of effectiveness should continue to be available.

Several publications have focused on the effectiveness of psychoanalytic approaches for depressed patients and have criticized the hegemony of CBT in this respect (Gabbard, Gunderson, & Fonagy, 2002; Leichsenring, Rabung, & Leibing, 2004). Even so, the all-too-frequent conflation of an underdeveloped evidence base for psychoanalytic interventions with a "weak" treatment prevails in the minds of those commissioning services. We will not rehearse these tensions here. Moreover, this external context is slowly showing signs of some change: in the United Kingdom, the Improving Access to Psychological Therapies Programme has now committed itself to an expansion in the range of psychological interventions on offer to patients beyond just CBT. Dynamic interpersonal therapy (DIT) has been adopted under the Programme as the "prototype" brief psychodynamic treatment option for depression.

The culture of evidence-based practice may be felt to be the "enemy", as it were, of psychoanalytic practice, but, as well as posing a threat, it has, in fact, helpfully focused our attention not only on the importance of systematically evaluating what we do so as to monitor the quality of what we offer to patients, but also on the thorny question of therapists' competence: how we define it, hone it, and assess it. In the United Kingdom, for example, the Department of Health has invested in the development of competences for a range of psychological therapies, including psychoanalytic psychotherapy, as the basis for the development of National Occupational Standards (NOS) for the practice of psychological therapies. The origins of DIT lie in this work. Before describing the model itself and its specific relevance for depressed patients, we will therefore briefly outline the competence framework that underpins the development of DIT. This paper is not intended to be clinical in its emphasis, as this is covered by Gelman, McKay, and Marks (2010) who describe their experience of implementing this model in their primary care service.

The rationale for developing DIT

The Improving Access to Psychological Therapies programme, launched in the United Kingdom in May 2007, provided the backdrop for the first wave of work on the development of competences for the practice of psychological therapies. The CBT competence model was specifically developed to be a "prototype" for articulating the competences associated with other psychological therapies (Roth & Pilling, 2008). The Psychoanalytic/Dynamic Competences Framework (Lemma, Roth, & Pilling, 2008),[1] which followed, describes a model of psychoanalytic/psychodynamic competences based on empirical evidence of efficacy. It indicates the various areas of activity that, taken together, represent what has been proven to be good clinical practice.

This work began with the identifying of those psychoanalytic/psychodynamic approaches with the strongest claims for evidence of efficacy, based on the outcome in controlled trials where a manual was available. In order to determine which studies to select, the reviews of psychological therapies conducted by Roth and Fonagy (2005) were combined with the trial and systematic review database held at the Centre for Outcomes, Research and Effectiveness, as part of scoping work for the National Institute for Health and Clinical Excellence (NICE). Working with the combined lists (in conjunction with an expert reference group comprising senior clinicians and researchers representative of different analytic traditions), clinical trials of appropriate quality for inclusion in the framework were identified, and the manuals used in these studies were located. Only those trials for which a manual could be accessed were included. These manuals were then studied carefully with a focus on what the therapists were expected to do. This qualitative analysis provided the basis for the articulation of the core, specific, and meta-competences required to practice psychoanalytic psychotherapy (see Figure 10.1). These competences were, where possible, peer-reviewed by the originators of the manuals and also by an expert reference group. To supplement these manuals, several widely cited texts that explicate psychoanalytic terminology and provide clear descriptions of how these concepts translate into clinical practice were also consulted (e.g. Bateman, Brown, & Pedder, 2000; Etchegoyen, 1999; Greenson, 1967; Lemma, 2003).

Because research trials monitor therapist performance through audio or video recordings that are then rated, we can be sure that therapists in these trials had adhered to the manual. This makes it possible to be reasonably confident that if procedures are followed as set out in the manual, which has been associated with substantial clinical improvements in research trials, there should be good outcomes for future patients also.

The core techniques and strategies underpinning DIT reflect the competences found to characterize models of psychoanalytic psychotherapy that have been shown to be effective (see Figure 10.1). In other words, DIT is based on a distillation of the evidence-based brief psychoanalytic/psychodynamic treatments pooled from the manualized approaches that were reviewed as part of this project. DIT deliberately uses methods taken from across the board of dynamic therapies, and we would therefore expect those who have been involved in the development of other brief dynamic models to find many familiar strategies and techniques in DIT.

New wine in an old bottle?

We are short neither of psychodynamic protocols nor of acronyms. In developing DIT (Lemma, Target, & Fonagy, 2011b) we did not wish to add to an already long list, and yet our experience as clinicians, trainers, and researchers persuaded us that the competence framework

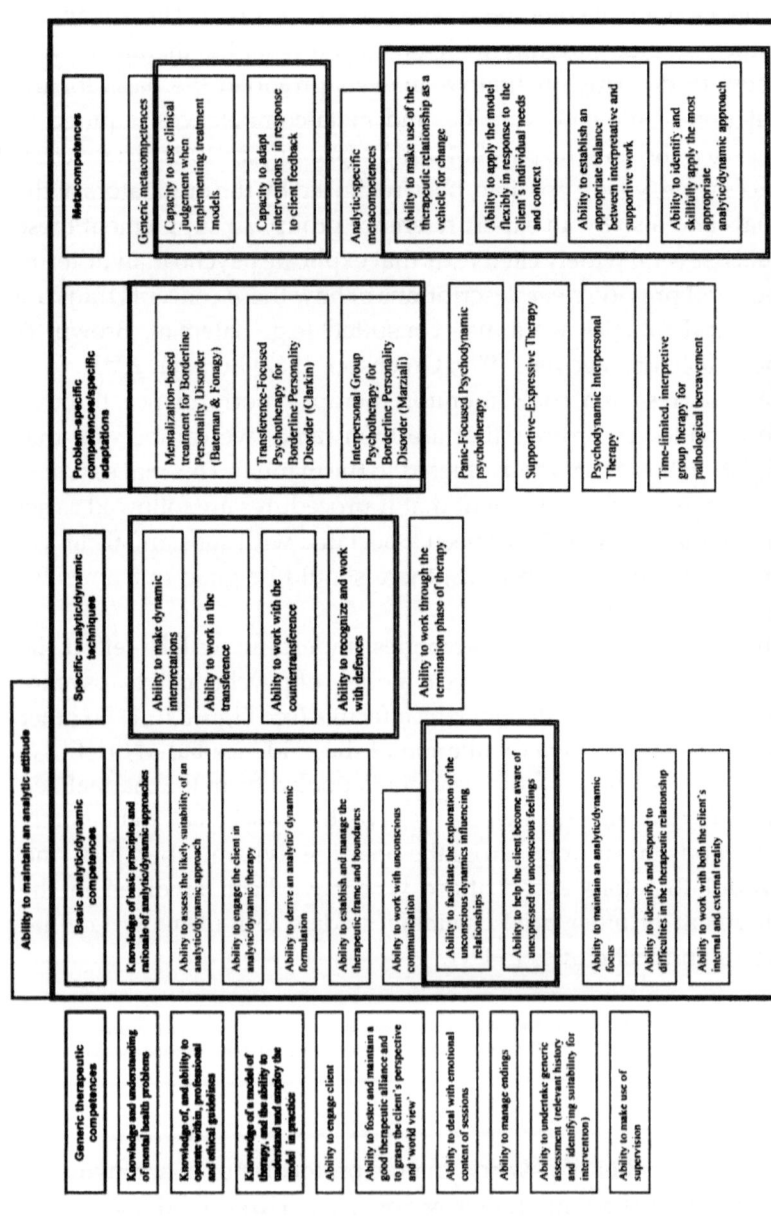

Figure 10.1. Map of psychoanalytic/dynamic competences.

228

provided an opportunity to develop a protocol that integrated core, shared analytic principles and techniques grounded in the extant evidence base and that would thus carry some external or empirical credibility when applied with a specific focus on depression.

Keeping the training burden to a minimum was one of the guiding principles for the development of this protocol. The different "versions" of brief psychodynamic therapy models that were examined as part of the development of the competence framework suggested that a variety of complex procedures are necessary to address the difficulties of specific patient populations—for example, borderline patients. However, many of these techniques, such as focusing primarily— even if by no means exclusively—on the transference relationship (Kernberg's transference-focused psychotherapy; Clarkin, Yeomans, & Kernberg, 2006), seemed too specialized for DIT. Nevertheless, the theories underpinning the manuals we consulted have greatly influenced the development and elaboration of the current protocol.

DIT was developed for pragmatic reasons, so that clinicians with a psychoanalytic/dynamic psychotherapy or counselling training can readily acquire the specific priorities and competences associated with time-limited therapeutic work (defined as 16 sessions in this model). This is a protocol that we have successfully piloted in a primary care context with consecutively referred depressed patients who were offered 16 sessions of DIT, as a basis for planning a larger-scale RCT. In all but one case, DIT was associated with a significant reduction in reported symptoms—to below clinical levels in 70% of the patients (Lemma, Target, & Fonagy, 2011a).

Feedback from both therapists and patients involved in the pilot study contributed to further refinement of the protocol. A four-day training, followed by weekly supervision of two video- or audiotaped cases, looks promising in its potential for helping dynamically oriented clinicians to achieve good results if they follow five relatively simple strategic steps in the course of a brief therapeutic engagement: (1) identify an attachment-related problem with a specific relational emotional focus that is felt by the patient to be currently making him[2] feel depressed; (2) work with the patient collaboratively to create an increasingly mentalistic picture of interpersonal issues raised by the problem; (3) encourage the patient to explore the possibility of alternative ways of feeling and thinking ("playing with a new internal and external reality"), actively using the transference relationship to bring to the fore the patient's characteristic ways of relating; (4) ensure that the therapeutic process (of change in self) is reflected on; and (5) near the end of treatment, present to the patient a written summary of the collaboratively created view of the person and the selected area of unconscious conflict, for him to hold on to, to reduce the risk of relapse (known to be very likely in clinical depression).

Although the techniques and strategies used in DIT reflect the findings of the broad competence framework for psychoanalytic psychotherapy, an approach that failed to contextualize theoretically what the therapist is aiming to do, and why, would be very limited. Consequently we have embedded DIT in a range of psychoanalytic ideas that we consider to be highly relevant to understanding depression and its impact on an individual's internal and external worlds, and which may give enough common ground to make the model of interest to psychoanalytic psychotherapists with a range of trainings; in particular, we drew on attachment theory, object relations theory, and Harry Stack Sullivan's interpersonal psychoanalysis (1968).

As is the case with other brief psychodynamically oriented approaches, in DIT the overarching principles are rooted in the broader psychoanalytic framework that emphasizes: (1) the impact of early childhood experiences on adult functioning, with particular attention to adult attachment processes and the significance of mental models of relationships; (2) the internal and external forces that shape the mind and therefore inform our perception of ourselves in relationships with others; (3) the existence of an unconscious realm of experience that is a motivating force; (4) the unconscious projective and introjective processes that underpin the subjective experience of relationships, and (5) the ubiquity of the transference, by which patients respond to others, and to the therapist, according to developmental models that have not been updated or challenged.

Why DIT for depression?

DIT formulates the presenting symptoms of depression as responses to interpersonal difficulties/perceived threats to attachments (loss/ separation) and hence also as threats to the self. DIT conceptualizes depression in terms of an underlying temporary disorganization of the attachment system caused by current relationship problems, which, in turn, generates a range of distortions in thinking and feelings typical of the depressive process. In the therapy a focus is maintained on this emotional "crisis" through an elaboration of the thoughts and feelings—conscious and unconscious—most characteristic of the particular patient and relevant to his depression, as these emerge in the context of the therapeutic relationship. Through the focused exploration of the transference relationship the patient is helped to develop a better understanding of his subjective reactions to threats. Making implicit anxieties and concerns explicit by improving the patient's ability to reflect on his own and other's thoughts and feelings, in turn, enhances the patient's ability to cope with current attachment-related interpersonal threats and challenges.

There are many features of depression that suggest that a dynamically oriented approach focusing on interpersonal issues is likely to be effective in addressing symptoms of major depression. Interpersonal problems are marked in severe depression and evident even in mild or moderate depression (Luyten, Corveleyn, & Blatt, 2005), driven not only by the potential of depressed mood to elicit negative responses from others, but also by those with depression being inclined to select and generate interpersonal scenarios with the propensity to evoke distress, such as conflicted interactions leading to social exclusion and rejection (see, for example, Kiesler, 1983; Lewinsohn, Mischel, Chaplin, & Barton, 1980).

The recent work of psychoanalytic researchers Sidney Blatt and Patrick Luyten demonstrates that not only is vulnerability to depression associated with the unconscious generation of interpersonal stress, but interpersonal factors explain much current data on the outcomes of treatments of depression (Blatt, Zuroff, Hawley, & Auerbach, in press; Luyten, Blatt, Van Houdenhove, & Corveleyn, 2006). There is increasing agreement in the field that the interpersonal aspects of depression should be given comparable weight to the normally highlighted intrapersonal dimensions (e.g. Hammen, 2005).

While the literature on distorted information processing in depression largely speaks to distortions of conscious cognition in depressed individuals (Beck, Rush, Shaw, & Emery, 1979; Kyte & Goodyer, 2008) some concepts in this literature, such as the dominance of a hopeless, helpless attributional style (Abramson, Seligman, & Teasdale, 1978) echo classical psychoanalytic writings that link these observations to unconscious projective and introjective processes (Engel & Schmale, 1967).

DIT as an approach specifically focuses on an individual's distorted and inadequate understanding of other people's thoughts and feelings. One aim of DIT is thus to enhance the patient's capacity to mentalize—an emphasis that is consistent with recently accumulating data demonstrating Theory of Mind deficits in patients with unipolar and bipolar depressive disorders (Inoue, Tonooka, Yamada, & Kanba, 2004; Inoue, Yamada, & Kanba, 2006; Kerr, Dunbar, & Bentall, 2003; Lee, Harkness, Sabbagh, & Jacobson, 2005; Montag et al., in press).

Measures of mentalizing in the attachment context also yield indications of a deficit associated with depression (Fischer-Kern et al., 2008; Fonagy et al., 1996; Müller, Kaufhold, Overbeck, & Grabhorn, 2006). This is important as DIT assumes failures of self- and other understanding in depression to be strongly tied to particular self–other interaction patterns evolved from childhood experiences, real or fantasized (see section below on the interpersonal affective focus).

Adaptive reflection or mentalization involves the integration of thinking and feeling, with a balance in focus between the two aspects such that realistic checking of assumptions can modulate mood and behaviour towards others. DIT aims to increase this capacity through the systematic work on one constellation of conscious and unconscious assumptions about self and others, and depressive reactions, most central for the patient at the time of referral; this work is described in greater detail below.

DIT has a dual focus on interpersonal and affective issues. The affective issues of greatest relevance centre on attachment-related concerns. Insecurely attached individuals are more likely to have more frequent depressive episodes and residual symptoms, use more pharmacotherapy, and be impaired in their social functioning (Conradi & de Jonge, 2009). There is a substantial body of work linking vulnerability to depression to insecure attachment (Bifulco, Moran, Ball, & Bernazzani, 2002; Bifulco, Moran, Ball, & Lillie, 2002; Grunebaum et al., in press; Lee & Hankin, 2009). Blatt's theory of depression in particular identifies two classes of attachment-history–based cognitive–affective schemata most likely to be found in depression: interpersonal dependency and excessive self-criticism (Blatt, 2008; Blatt & Luyten, 2009) linked to preoccupied and avoidant patterns of attachment, respectively (Blatt & Luyten, 2009).

Core features of DIT

The DIT therapist has two aims: (1) to help the patient to understand the connection between his presenting symptoms and what is happening in his relationships by identifying a core, unconscious, repetitive pattern of relating that becomes the focus of the therapy; (2) to try to enhance the patient's capacity to reflect on his own states of mind and so enhance his ability to manage interpersonal difficulties.

This model, along with the majority of brief psychodynamic models, can be conceptualized as consisting of three phases: an engagement/assessment phase (Sessions 1–4), a middle phase (Sessions 5–12), and an ending phase (Sessions 13–16), each with its own distinctive strategies.

The interpersonal–affective focus (IPAF)

The primary task of the initial phase, which organizes DIT's therapeutic thrust, then follows, which is typically to identity one dominant and recurring unconscious interpersonal pattern that is meaningfully connected with the onset and/or maintenance of the depressive symptoms. We understand this pattern as being underpinned by a particular representation of self-in-relation-to-an-other that characterizes the patient's interpersonal style and that leads to difficulties in his relationships because of the way it organizes his interpersonal behaviour. These representations are typically linked to a particular affect(s) and defensive manouevres. Affects are understood to be responses to the activation, in the patient's mind, of a specific self–other representation. Kernberg's (1980) integration of object relations theory with ego psychology in the theoretical frame of transference-focused psychotherapy (Clarkin, Yeomans, & Kernberg, 2006) is very close to the heart of DIT's theoretical basis and way of formulating a focus for the intervention.

Past experiences, while clearly informing current functioning and internal object relations, are not the major focus of the DIT. They are included in the formulation shared with the patient so as to meaningfully frame his current difficulties in the context of his lived experience over time, but they are not a central component of the therapeutic process. Rather, given the brief nature of the therapy, the focus is on a core segment of the patients' interpersonal functioning that is closely connected with the presenting symptom(s). The therapist identifies the most important current and past relationships but does so with emphasis on present. The relationships brought to the assessment are characterized according to considerations born of attachment theory primarily as a heuristic device. The therapist strives to establish the form of a relationship, the key processes employed in maintaining it, whether it has changed over time, and how it relates to problems—whether, for example, it makes depression worse.

The IPAF guides the therapist's interventions during the middle phase of the therapy (Sessions 5–12). During this phase the therapist helps the patient to stay focused on, and work through, the IPAF and to try out new, more adaptive ways of resolving his interpersonal difficulties. A consistent effort is made to encourage and support the patient to make psychological sense of what is happening in his own mind, in others' minds, and in important interactions. The last four sessions (13–16) are devoted to helping the patient to explore the affective experience and unconscious meaning of ending the therapy, to review progress, and to help him to anticipate future difficulties/vulnerabilities.

Case illustration:
Arriving at an IPAF

Marc, a man in his mid-twenties, was referred by his GP after he was signed him off work for two consecutive weeks due to stress at work with his boss. Marc explained that he had never taken to his boss because he was "loud" and "brash". A few months prior to being signed off work by his GP, Marc had felt particularly humiliated by his boss after he was openly critical of one of Marc's reports in front of other colleagues. At the time, Marc had barely spoken, feeling himself immediately to be "stupid". Subsequently, he felt that everyone viewed him differently, and he found it increasingly hard to even look people in the eye when he was at work. He ruminated over this exchange in his mind, and the more he did so, the more angry he became. He spoke about the "injustice" of it all, as he was hard-working and diligent.

As Marc spoke about his difficulties, the therapist (AL) became aware that he was having a particular impact on her: she felt she was being recruited into siding with Marc against the boss, who had become the personification of evil. The therapist made a mental note of this but said nothing at this stage. This feeling nevertheless grew stronger as he described his relationship with his younger brother in more detail.

Marc was the older of two. His father had died unexpectedly of a heart attack when he was 5 years old. Following the father's death, his mother appeared to have sunk into a very depressed state of mind from which she never fully emerged. Marc still lived at home with his mother, while his younger brother left home to move in with his girlfriend. He felt that his brother had acted selfishly, leaving home just when Marc had taken up his new job and their mother had become more severely depressed. Consequently, Marc had felt that the burden of care for his mother had fallen on him, as he felt it always had done since his father's death.

The description of his brother bore an uncanny similarity to Marc's hated boss. His brother was described as loud, unthinking, and selfish. They had never been close, and he reluctantly acknowledged that his brother was very successful in life. He spontaneously recounted that as they were only 18 months apart, they had shared many friends and gone to the same school, but that he felt he was always in his brother's shadow because of the latter's more outgoing personality. When the therapist invited him to elaborate on this, Marc gave a very detailed account of his brother's superior physical achievements. In this respect he thought that his brother had taken after their father, who had been an excellent runner in his time. He added somewhat pointedly that his brother had been fortunate to inherit his father's height and strength, whereas he had followed in the maternal footsteps: his mother's family was described as a family of "clever thinkers prone to depression".

Marc said he did not really feel that he knew his father, except through his mother's "rose-tinted glasses". He had grown up hearing what an impressive character he had been, and he mentioned twice the way his mother referred to the father's "stature" both concretely, as he had indeed been tall and strong, and because of his standing in the world of work. As Marc spoke, he conveyed a sense of hopelessness about his own capacity to be impressive, and the therapist reflected this back to him.

By the end of Session 2, the therapist had become conscious of a pattern in the room: whenever she tried to be empathic or made some observation, Marc either seemed to ignore it or typically replied that "it was not quite like that". The therapist began to feel that she was being carefully scrutinized and duly criticized, as if in the room the roles had been reversed: it was now Marc who was in some way criticizing her reports, just as he reported his boss had done to him.

In Session 3, the therapist explored further the circumstances around the time when Marc's brother had left home. It became clear that the onset of a more insidious state of depression dated back to that time, and that it had been further aggravated by the more recent incidents at work. It emerged that the mother had felt bereft by the brother's decision to move away from the family home. She appeared to have been stuck in an unresolved grief reaction following the death of her husband, which was fuelled with new impetus by the departure of her younger son. All this appeared to have deeply angered Marc, who had seemingly always felt in the shadow of his father's and brother's greater stature in his mother's eyes. The incident at work had been the final blow for him as he had somehow always managed to reassure himself of his superior intellect as a defence against his deep-rooted conviction that he was simply not good enough for his mother. To be attacked publicly—as he saw it—for producing a bad report reduced his intellectual stature, and he felt profoundly humiliated and exposed to the critical eyes of others. His anxiety had, indeed, a distinctly paranoid flavour. His basic response to this interpersonal scenario was one of passive aggression, where he said nothing, withdrew into himself, and internally remained locked in a grievance against the other person. His most profound grievance was towards the parental couple in his mind, by whom he felt painfully excluded.

In approaching a possible focus, the therapist began by summarizing the way Marc had conveyed to her his long-standing experience of not having any stature in his mother's eyes, and that this characterized more generally his expectation of how other people viewed him. She acknowledged the importance to him of his intellectual pursuits as a way of reassuring himself and others that he did have substance and stature in his own right. Consequently, work had been overvalued such that it had not only pulled him away from developing relationships, but it had also made him highly sensitive to any slight to his intellect.

The therapist spoke with Marc about the heavy burden of having to bear not just the meaning for him of the early loss of his father but, perhaps even more significantly, to have to nurse his mother through her ongoing sense of loss, which he could never assuage. He seemed to feel that he had lived in the shadow of his father and brother, both of whom had managed to escape the fate of the "clever thinkers prone to depression", leaving him feeling as if he was forever lagging behind them in some fundamental way, which nothing could change. At the same time he was having to take care of a mother who both needed him but also made him feel second-best.

Marc replied by emphasizing that in the intellectual domain he had always shone, but that somehow this was never really valued, even though he had always thought that his mother, herself an academic, prized intelligence. The therapist observed that he seemed always to have been very preoccupied with what his mother was looking for, and that he felt confused about what she valued and admired. His whole life, in a way, had been devoted to getting it right for his mother rather than for himself.

She then wondered with him whether now that they were negotiating what to work on in therapy, he might be similarly preoccupied with what he imagined the therapist would prize. This appeared to resonate with Marc, who observed how anxious he had felt each time he had come for the session. He then reported a dream he had had the night before the third session, in which *he had been jeered at by a group of adolescents.* In the dream *he wanted to shout back, but no words came out.*

By this stage the therapist felt confident enough to propose an IPAF. She suggested that a recurring experience for Marc in his relationships was to feel that he was small, lacking in stature, insufficient, while the other person was more typically either explicitly humiliating and rejecting (as he had felt his boss had been recently) or implicitly humiliating (as he felt his mother had been, leaving him feeling that he could never live up to his father's/brother's stature). His only option seemed to be to follow on in the maternal family tradition of "clever thinkers prone to depression". Distressing though this was, the therapist suggested that this way Marc at least comforted himself with a likeness to his mother, which he felt only he shared with her.

At this stage the therapist did not share her hypothesis that Marc also took up the position of being the critical one in his own mind and subjected the other to harsh scrutiny, because she considered that this would be too much for him to take on board at this point and might, indeed, make him feel criticized by her. However, this would be an important theme that was further elaborated during the middle phase of therapy.

Here-and-now focus

DIT maintains a focus on the patient's interpersonal functioning in the here-and-now of his current life and of the therapeutic session. The here-and-now focus is central to DIT and denotes three related activities:

First, it refers to the focus on what the patient is *currently* feeling in the session. This requires careful tracking of the patient's emotional state during the session, so as to communicate an understanding of this to the patient in order to help him to recognize his feelings as his own, differentiate feelings from actions, and allow discussion of the connections between feelings and actions, which facilitates self-understanding and awareness of motivations attributed to others—for example: "I missed last week's session because when I feel anxious I want to avoid being with you—because I think you find me boring and hopeless."

Second, it refers to a primary focus on the exploration of *current* difficulties in the patient's life rather than on trying to establish links to the childhood origins of these difficulties. This way the patient can be helped to feel he is working on difficulties that are live and current and over which he can effect a degree of change.

Third—and related to the above points—it refers to the active use of the patient–therapist relationship to help the patient to explore the IPAF in the immediacy of the transference relationship.

Focus on the patient's mind

A distinguishing feature of DIT is that it approaches the exploration of problematic interpersonal patterns not by addressing the patient's behaviour, but through its consistent focus on the patient's mental states—beliefs, feelings, wishes, and thoughts—in themselves and in others. A primary aim is to provide the patient with an experience of being with another person who is interested in *thinking with* the patient about what distresses him so as to stimulate the patient's own capacity for reflecting on his own experience.

This is what we label the collaborative stance the DIT therapist must establish with her patient. The goal is not simply to work on an unconscious conflict; rather, the aim is primarily to use the patient's reports of his interpersonal experiences as a way of helping him to develop his own capacity for thinking and feeling his experience. This focus is fundamental to DIT, and it informs technique insofar as the helpfulness of the therapist's interventions—such as the interpretation of transference—is evaluated against the criterion of whether they help to stimulate the patient's capacity to reflect on their own subjective experience in relation to that of others, in the context of a problematic interpersonal relationship.

The DIT therapist is particularly interested in making explicit what has effectively become procedural so that the patient is then better able to effect change in how he manages his relationships. Working through the IPAF therefore involves enhancing the patient's awareness of how his behaviour is driven by mental states. The aim is to review the experience related to the IPAF as much in the present as possible—what the patient feels right now. The patient's phenomenal experience is explored in the relational realm, not just the intrapersonal one.

Therapeutic stance

The DIT therapist adopts an involved, empathic manner. The aim is to work collaboratively with the patient from the outset, especially in arriving at a formulation that provides a meaningful focus for the patient. The therapist is explicit about her understanding of the patient's problems, openly discussing and checking out the formulation with the patient and jointly elaborating it in their formulation statement. The aim is to create the opportunity for the patient to actively participate in agreeing and understanding a focus for the work.

The therapist is receptive to the patient's feedback. If the patient questions the therapist's understanding or her perception of the treatment, the therapist responds non-defensively, providing a clear, unambiguous account of how she has arrived at her understanding. The aim is to be as transparent as possible while being attuned to, and working with, the patient's need, where it arises, to control the therapist through projective processes.

The therapist strives to adopt a "not-knowing" but curious stance that prioritizes the joint exploration of the patient's mental states as they relate to the identified interpersonal process that has been agreed on as the focus of the therapy. Interpretations of deep unconscious material are generally avoided in favour of the facilitation and support of the patient's own capacity to stand back from his own immediate experience in order to be able to reflect on it.

Although the basic stance is a psychoanalytic one, rooted in an interest in the patient's unconscious communications and in making use of the transference, the brevity of the treatment requires more activity on the part of the therapist.

Techniques

In DIT the therapist intervenes to generate, clarify, and elaborate interpersonally relevant information. A key intervention is to help the patient to stay focused on the agreed IPAF. All the techniques used support this core aim—that is, of helping the patient to better understand what is happening for him, in his mind, when things go wrong in his relationships, including how the IPAF is enacted in the therapeutic relationship. To this end, DIT draws liberally on supportive and expressive techniques while also making judicious use of directive techniques to support change within a brief time frame.

No therapy can occur without some *supportive* techniques: support and empathy are necessary components of all therapies, and the therapeutic skills of reflective listening and accurate empathy are a fundamental aspect of DIT. This does not mean that the therapist agrees with everything the patient says. Confrontation or challenge is an equally important aspect of DIT.

Because DIT is used with patients whose depression ranges from mild to severe and may sometimes be co-morbid with Axis II disorders, the therapist needs to titrate the level of supportive interventions offered to a given patient. The less impaired patient, with a higher level of pre-morbid interpersonal functioning, is more likely to make greater use of expressive techniques without requiring more supportive interventions to bolster defences and support his day-to-day functioning. The ability to apply the model flexibly and to balance supportive and expressive techniques is therefore essential.

The *expressive* techniques used in DIT will be familiar to all analytically trained clinicians: clarification, confrontation, and interpretation. Particular emphasis is placed on identifying and helping the patient to reflect on unverbalized feelings. As with all analytic approaches, the therapist considers the possible meaning of her own emotional reactions to the patient a basis for facilitating this exploration.

As would be the case in any analytic therapy, the therapist will make judicious use of silence so as to allow the emergence of the patient's uninterrupted flow of associations and communications. However, given the brevity of the treatment, the DIT therapist is far more active than when practising longer term analytic therapy, guided by DIT's focus on helping the patient to actively start working on his difficulties within the brief time frame of the therapy.

This greater activity does not usually involve giving advice, but it requires that the therapist is alert to any deviations from the agreed focus so as to re-direct the patient back to the focus. It also requires that the therapist explicitly support the patient's attempts to change. To this extent some *directive* techniques are used during the middle phase of treatment. Such interventions include asking questions more freely to clarify the patient's experience and active encouragement to try out different ways of approaching a conflict with another person. They are considered to have a subtle structuring impact on the patient's perspective on his experience.

The way directive techniques are deployed in DIT is nevertheless framed in the context of a good understanding of the meaning that the therapist's more directive stance may acquire for the patient in light of the IPAF. For example, an anxious patient for whom separation is felt to be terrifying may well be very compliant with the therapist's direction, because non-compliance is felt to be a threat to the relationship. Yet, in spite of the therapist's support and encouragement, little change takes place in this patient. In such an instance, the DIT therapist would be attuned to the unconscious meaning that may be latent in the patient's wish to please the therapist and would actively address this with the patient, linking it to the identified IPAF and the lack of progress in the therapy.

Working in the transference

Transference interpretations are used to support the aim of helping the patient to identify the implicit representations of himself and others that underpin his problematic interpersonal patterns—that is, the IPAF. The therapist actively encourages the patient to discuss and explore his perceptions of, and feelings about, the therapist and how he thinks the therapist may feel or think about him. The aim is to help the patient to explore the IPAF in his relationship to the therapist, making links and drawing parallels between his subjective experience with others outside the therapy—people past and present, *but especially with those currently in the patient's life*—and with the therapist (and vice versa).

In DIT the primary aim of a transference interpretation is not to arrive at an insight; rather, the goal is to engage the patient in the process of making sense of how his mind works. Using what happens in the transference provides the most immediate way of doing this.

By virtue of the brief nature of the therapy, transference interpretations are used in a more circumscribed manner than in longer term analytic therapies. A transference interpretation is made primarily because it enhances the exploration of the IPAF, or because it is needed to help the overall working alliance—for example, if there seems to be a danger that the patient will drop out of therapy because of a transference fantasy that the therapist wants to get rid of him. This may or may not be part of the chosen IPAF.

The use of outcome-monitoring measures

One of the features of this protocol, partly dictated by its intended use within IAPT services, is the inclusion of session-by-session outcome monitoring—a demand that is unfamiliar to many psychoanalytic therapists. As a part of DIT, therapists administer measures at the start of each session. Although this practice is often anticipated to be intrusive to the therapeutic process, in our experience this is typically an intrusion felt more acutely by the therapist than by the patient.

This monitoring, as well as providing both patient and therapist with another form of feedback on how the patient is feeling week-to-week, also often brings to the fore areas of "stuckness" or resistance. Once the therapist is acculturated to the routine of outcome monitoring, the "use" made of the questionnaires by the patient becomes grist to the therapeutic mill and is integrated into the therapeutic process. For example, one patient reported significant improvement in the sessions, yet her scores on the questionnaires remained very high. When this discrepancy was taken up by the therapist, it made it possible to understand, at the level of the transference, the patient's wish to "punish" the therapist and deprive her of evidence she might share with others that the therapy was of help—an enactment of the grievance the patient harboured towards her mother.

While our experience of supervising clinicians using DIT has persuaded us that outcome monitoring can be usefully integrated into routine practice, we also recognize that the measures used within IAPT services do not meaningfully capture the kind of change that DIT attempts to promote. This is something we intend to address eventually in a larger scale RCT.

Conclusion

DIT is not a new approach as such; rather, it reflects our attempt to integrate the empirically supported aspects of psychodynamic therapy into a coherent model that is relatively easy to acquire by professionals already trained in psychodynamic therapy or counselling, and that can be delivered within a public health sector setting.

The initial and very preliminary pilot study we carried out demonstrated that this model was easy to grasp and implement by clinicians who had not undergone an intensive analytic training, but who were experienced at offering once-weekly psychodynamic therapy in the NHS. The qualitative data obtained from the patients also suggested that the approach was felt to be congenial and relevant to their presenting concerns. A large-scale RCT is now under way to determine the value of this particular application of psychodynamic ideas to the treatment of depression.

Notes

This chapter is based on a substantially modified version of: A. Lemma, M. Target, & P. Fonagy, "The Development of a Brief Psychodynamic Protocol for Depression: Dynamic Interpersonal Therapy (DIT)", *Psychoanalytic Psychotherapy*, 24 (4, 2010): 329–346 (http://www.informaworld.com). This development has resulted from a collaboration between the Tavistock and Portman NHS Foundation Trust and the Anna Freud Centre.

1. The full list of competences can be accessed at www.ucl.ac.uk/CORE
2. For clarity and economy, the patient is referred to throughout the chapter as "he" and the therapist as "she".

References

Abramson, L. Y., Seligman, M. E. P., & Teasdale, J. D. (1978). Learned helplessness in humans: Critique and reformulation. *Journal of Abnormal Psychology, 87*: 49–74.

Angst, J., & Dobler-Mikola, A. (1985). The Zurich Study. VI. A continuum from depression to anxiety disorders? *European Archives of Psychiatry and Neurological Science, 235*: 179–186.

Bateman, A., Brown, D., & Pedder, J. (2000). *Introduction to Psychotherapy: An Outline of Psychodynamic Principles and Practice* (3rd edition). London: Routledge.

Beck, A. T., Rush, J., Shaw, B., & Emery, G. (1979). *Cognitive Therapy of Depression*. New York: Guilford Press.

Bifulco, A., Moran, P. M., Ball, C., & Bernazzani, O. (2002). Adult attachment style. I: Its relationship to clinical depression. *Social Psychiatry & Psychiatric Epidemiology, 37*: 50–59.

Bifulco, A., Moran, P. M., Ball, C., & Lillie, A. (2002). Adult attachment style. II: Its relationship to psychosocial depressive-vulnerability. *Social Psychiatry & Psychiatric Epidemiology, 37*: 60–67.

Blatt, S. J. (2008). *Polarities of Experience: Relatedness and Self Definition in Personality Development, Psychopathology, and the Therapeutic Process.* Washington, DC: American Psychological Association.

Blatt, S. J., & Luyten, P. (2009). A structural–developmental psychodynamic approach to psychopathology: Two polarities of experience across the life span. *Development and Psychopathology, 21* (3), 793–814.

Blatt, S. J., Zuroff, D. C., Hawley, L. L., & Auerbach, J. S. (in press). Predictors of sustained therapeutic change. *Psychotherapy Research.*

Clarkin, J., Yeomans, F., & Kernberg, O. (2006). *Psychotherapy for Borderline Personality: Focusing on Object Relations*. Washington, DC: American Psychiatric Press.

Conradi, H. J., & de Jonge, P. (2009). Recurrent depression and the role of adult attachment: A prospective and a retrospective study. *Journal of Affective Disorders, 116* (1–2): 93–99.

Eaton, W., Shao, H., Nesdadt, G., Lee, B., Bienvenu, O., & Zandi, P. (2008). Population-based study of first onset and chronicity in major depressive disorder. *Archives of General Psychiatry, 65*: 513–520.

Engel, G. L., & Schmale, A. H., Jr. (1967). Psychoanalytic theory of somatic disorder: Conversion, specificity, and the disease onset situation. *Journal of the American Psychoanalytic Association, 15*: 344–365.

Etchegoyen, R. H. (1999). *Fundamentals of Psychoanalytic Technique* (revised edition). London: Karnac.

Fischer-Kern, M., Tmej, A., Kapusta, N. D., Naderer, A., Leithner-Dziubas, K., Löffler-Stastka, H., et al. (2008). Mentalisierungsfähigkeit bei depressiven Patientinnen: Eine Pilotstudie. *Zeitschrift für Psychosomatische Medizin und Psychotherapie, 54*: 368–380.

Fonagy, P. (2010). The changing shape of clinical practice: A comprehensive narrative review. *Psychoanalytic Psychotherapy, 24* (1): 22–43.

Fonagy, P., Leigh, T., Steele, M., Steele, H., Kennedy, R., Mattoon, G., et al. (1996). The relation of attachment status, psychiatric classification, and response to psychotherapy. *Journal of Consulting and Clinical Psychology, 64*: 22–31.

Gabbard, G. O., Gunderson, J. G., & Fonagy, P. (2002). The place of psychoanalytic treatments within psychiatry. *Archives of General Psychiatry, 59*: 505–510.

Gelman, T., McKay, A., & Marks, L. (2010). Dynamic Interpersonal Therapy: Providing a focus for time-limited psychodynamic work within the NHS. *Psychoanalytic Psychotherapy: Applications, Theory and Research, 24* (4): 347–361.

Goldberg, D. (2009). The interplay between biological and psychological factors in determining vulnerability to mental disorders. *Psychoanalytic Psychotherapy, 23* (3): 236–247.

Greenson, R. R. (1967). *The Technique and Practice of Psychoanalysis, Vol. 1*. New York: International Universities Press.

Grunebaum, M. F., Galfalvy, H. C., Mortenson, L. Y., Burke, A. K., Oquendo, M. A., & Mann, J. J. (in press). Attachment and social adjustment: Relationships to suicide attempt and major depressive episode in a prospective study. *Journal of Affective Disorders*.

Hammen, C. (2005). Stress and depression. *Annual Review of Clinical Psychology, 1* (1): 293–319.

Inoue, Y., Tonooka, Y., Yamada, K., & Kanba, S. (2004). Deficiency of theory of mind in patients with remitted mood disorder. *Journal of Affective Disorders, 82* (3): 403–409.

Inoue, Y., Yamada, K., & Kanba, S. (2006). Deficit in theory of mind is a risk for relapse of major depression. *Journal of Affective Disorders, 95* (1–3): 125–127.

Kernberg, O. (1980). *Internal World and External Reality: Object Relations Theory Applied.* New York: Jason Aronson.

Kerr, N., Dunbar, R. I. M., & Bentall, R. P. (2003). Theory of mind deficits in bipolar affective disorder. *Journal of Affective Disorders, 73* (3): 253–259.

Kessler, R. C., Berglund, P., Demler, O., Jin, R., Koretz, D., Merikangas, K. R., et al. (2003). The epidemiology of major depressive disorder: Results from the National Comorbidity Survey Replication (NCS-R). *Journal of the American Medical Association, 289*: 3095–3105.

Kiesler, D. J. (1983). The 1982 interpersonal circle: A taxonomy for complementarity in human transactions. *Psychological Review, 90*: 185–214.

Kupfer, D. J. (1991). Long-term treatment of depression. *Journal of Clinical Psychiatry, 52* (Suppl. 5): 28–34.

Kyte, Z. A., & Goodyer, I. (2008). Social cognition in depressed children and adolescents. In C. Sharp, P. Fonagy, & I. Goodyer (Eds.), *Social Cognition and Developmental Psychopathology* (pp. 201–237). Oxford: Oxford University Press.

Lee, A., & Hankin, B. L. (2009). Insecure attachment, dysfunctional attitudes, and low self-esteem predicting prospective symptoms of depression and anxiety during adolescence. *Journal of Clinical Child and Adolescent Psychology, 38* (2): 219–231.

Lee, L., Harkness, K. L., Sabbagh, M. A., & Jacobson, J. A. (2005). Mental state decoding abilities in clinical depression. *Journal of Affective Disorders, 86* (2–3): 247–258.

Leichsenring, F., Rabung, S., & Leibing, E. (2004). The efficacy of short-term psychodynamic psychotherapy in specific psychiatric disorders: A meta-analysis. *Archives of General Psychiatry, 61*: 1208–1216.

Lemma, A. (2003). *Introduction to the Practice of Psychoanalytic Psychotherapy.* Chichester: John Wiley.

Lemma, A., Roth, A., & Pilling, S. (2008). *The Competences Required to Deliver Effective Psychoanalytic/Psychodynamic Therapy.* Available at: www.ucl.ac.uk/CORE

Lemma, A., Target, M., & Fonagy, P. (2011a). The development of a brief psychodynamic intervention (Dynamic Interpersonal Therapy) and its application to depression: A pilot study. *Psychiatry: Biological and Interpersonal Processes, 74* (1): 43–50.

Lemma, A., Target, M., & Fonagy, P. (2011b). *Dynamic Interpersonal Therapy: A Clinician's Guide.* Oxford: Oxford University Press.

Lewinsohn, P. M., Mischel, W., Chaplin, W., & Barton, R. (1980). Social competence and depression: The role of illusory self-perception. *Journal of Abnormal Psychology, 89:* 203–212.

Luyten, P., Blatt, S. J., Van Houdenhove, B., & Corveleyn, J. (2006). Depression research and treatment: Are we skating to where the puck is going to be? *Clinical Psychology Review, 26* (8): 985–999.

Luyten, P., Corveleyn, J., & Blatt, S. J. (2005). The convergence among psychodynamic and cognitive–behavioral theories of depression: A critical overview of empirical research. In: J. Corveleyn, P. Luyten, & S. J. Blatt (Eds.), *The Theory and Treatment of Depression: Towards a Dynamic Interactionism Model* (pp. 107–147). Mahwah, NJ: Lawrence Erlbaum Associates.

Malhi, G., Adams, P., Porter, R., Wignall, A, Lampe, L., O'Connor, N., et al. (2009). Clinical practice recommendations for depression. *Acta Psychiatrica Scandinavica, 119* (Suppl. 439): 8–26.

Moffitt, T. E., Harrington, H., Caspi, A., Kim-Cohen, J., Goldberg, D., Gregary, A. M., et al. (2007). Depression and generalized anxiety disorder: Cumulative and sequential comorbidity in a birth cohort followed prospectively to age 32 years. *Archives of General Psychiatry, 64* (5): 651–660.

Montag, C., Ehrlich, A., Neuhaus, K., Dziobek, I., Heekeren, H. R., Heinz, A., et al. (in press). Theory of mind impairments in euthymic bipolar patients. *Journal of Affective Disorders.*

Müller, C., Kaufhold, J., Overbeck, G., & Grabhorn, R. (2006). The importance of reflective functioning to the diagnosis of psychic structure. *Psychology and Psychotherapy, 79* (4): 485–494.

Roth, A. D., & Fonagy, P. (2005). *What Works for Whom? A Critical Review of Psychotherapy Research* (2nd edition). New York: Guilford Press.

Roth, A. D., & Pilling, S. (2008). Using an evidence-based methodology to identify the competences required to deliver effective cognitive and behavioural therapy for depression and anxiety disorders. *Behavioural and Cognitive Psychotherapy, 36:* 129–147.

Sullivan, H. S. (1968). *The Interpersonal Theory of Psychiatry.* New York: W. W. Norton.

Taylor, D. (2009). Consenting to be robbed so as not to be murdered. *Psychoanalytic Psychotherapy*, 23 (4): 263–275.

Ustun, T., Ayuso-Mateos, J., Chatterji, S., Mathers, C., & Murray, C. (2004). Global burden of depressive disorders in the year 2000+. *British Journal of Psychiatry*, 184: 386–392.

Westen, D., Novotny, C. M., & Thompson-Brenner, H. (2004). The empirical status of empirically supported psychotherapies: Assumptions, findings, and reporting in controlled clinical trials. *Psychological Bulletin*, 130: 631–663.

INDEX